PSYCHOTHERAPEUTIC DRUGS

Publication Number 350

AMERICAN LECTURE SERIES®

A Monograph in

The BANNERSTONE DIVISION *of*

AMERICAN LECTURES IN DERMATOLOGY

Edited by

ARTHUR C. CURTIS, M.D.

Chairman, Department of Dermatology and Syphilology
University of Michigan
Ann Arbor, Michigan

PSYCHOTHERAPEUTIC DRUGS

By

ASHTON L. WELSH, M.S., M.D.

Assistant Professor of Dermatology and Syphilology
University of Cincinnati, College of Medicine
Cincinnati, Ohio

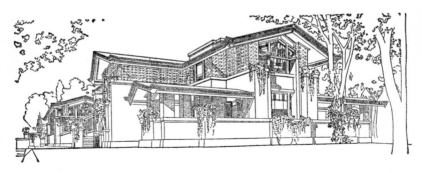

CHARLES C THOMAS • PUBLISHER
Springfield · Illinois · U.S.A.

CHARLES C THOMAS · PUBLISHER
BANNERSTONE HOUSE
301-327 East Lawrence Avenue, Springfield, Illinois, U.S.A.

Published simultaneously in the British Commonwealth of Nations by
BLACKWELL SCIENTIFIC PUBLICATIONS, LTD., OXFORD, ENGLAND

Published simultaneously in Canada by
THE RYERSON PRESS, TORONTO

Library of Congress Catalog Card Number: 58-14080

With THOMAS BOOKS *careful attention is given to all details
of manufacturing and design. It is the Publisher's desire to
present books that are satisfactory as to their physical qualities
and artistic possibilities and appropriate for their particular use.*
THOMAS BOOKS *will be true to those laws of quality that
assure a good name and good will.*

Printed in the United States of America

To members of the medical profession
this volume is dedicated
for the better service of Humanity

FOREWORD

Preparation of this monograph was undertaken for the purpose of bringing together, within the covers of one book, important information about certain psychotherapeutic agents for which tranquilization, ataraxia, or "peace of mind" has been claimed.

The introduction of a multiplicity of psychotherapeutic drugs, and of new terms, such as tranquilizer, ataraxic, normalizer, calmative, neurosedative, neuroleptic, psychic energizer, pacific, antiphobic and phrenotropic has created a difficult situation. Physicians are confronted with the problem of evaluating claims of usefulness for a wide variety of chemical substances with diverse pharmacological effects, which are proposed for the treatment of neurotic and psychic disorders. It appears probable that the gradually increasing number of new drugs, as well as new terms, will add to, rather than detract from, the confusion.

The message which it is my wish to convey in the pages of this monograph can best be expressed by direct quotation from a Report of the Council on Drugs, which appeared in the *Journal of the American Medical Association*, March 1, 1958:[277]

> "It seems wise to bear in mind that regardless of terminology, the ideal objective of psychotherapy with drugs is to induce an improved mental state, irrespective of what subjective symptom or objective sign is being treated. This should be done with agents that produce no undesirable subjective responses, are lacking in toxic side actions, and exert no summative effects with other drugs unless the latter are beneficial."

ASHTON L. WELSH, M. D.

Cincinnati, Ohio

PREFACE

In the United States, the consumption of psychotherapeutic drugs for tranquilization, or ataraxia of the human mental state, or for "peace of mind," has soared at an alarming rate since the hesitant introduction of such medicaments in 1954. According to some reports, in total sales, tranquilizers are exceeded only by antibiotics and vitamins. Consequently, the production and marketing of ataractic drugs has become typical American "Big Business."

Some of these drugs have undergone intensive investigation and have received much publicity. The word "tranquilizer" has been accorded an honored place in newspapers, lay publications, in advertising and entertainment media, with the result that there is an unparalleled demand on the members of the medical profession for what appears to be a panacea, with which to reduce the morbidity of psychoneurotic illness. Such demand is merely a reflection of stress imposed by contemporary civilization.

We might well pause to consider the implications of mass dependency on psychotherapeutic agents for tranquilization, on "peace pills," because many of these agents are relatively untried and unpredictable. In many of them lie, for the patient, physical danger, as well as alteration of life processes with physical changes.

Traditionally, the psychiatrist was a clinician, and not a researcher in the field of therapeutic investigation. Necessary requirements imposed upon the pharmaceutical suppliers for clinical trials of their products soon overtaxed the psychiatrists, and the inevitable result has been hurried, uncontrolled, sometimes misleading reporting in the medical literature, by physicians in every field of medicine. Although many ataractic agents may show promise, and we welcome their appearance, conservative clinical use commensurate with current status is desirable.

There are few well-controlled studies on the use of the newer tranquilizing agents, and there is even scanty laboratory information about their pharmacologic properties. Since the cerebral cortex is relatively inaccessible, there are no accurate, useful screening methods for determining the actions of these drugs. Widespread use of these new drugs does not seem justified, on the basis of the dearth of clinical reports.

A few years ago, when a dermatologist questioned a patient for the first time concerning adherence, if any, to some internal therapeutic regimen, the patient, who was already receiving more-or-less familiar therapy for specific illnesses, was the exception rather than the rule. Today, dermatologists in various parts of the country report that almost every patient is on tranquilizing therapy, by the time of the first dermatological consultation. In my own experience, one of the first questions which I have learned to ask new patients concerns such therapy. In response to my query, I find that just about half of those patients are either taking a tranquilizing drug or have taken one or more of such drugs.

Diagnosis of manifestations of reaction to psychotherapeutic drugs has become a problem which the dermatologist must solve— daily. During the past four years, I have encountered a number of diagnoses wherein I failed, or nearly failed, to recognize that a given dermatosis might be the result of untoward reaction to a tranquilizing drug. Until World War II, physicians were indoctrinated with the concept that "syphilis is the Great Imitator," and that for the welfare of the patient a high "index of suspicion" must be maintained. The dermatologist of today sees, rarely, a patient with active syphilis; there is no longer need to maintain such "index of suspicion" regarding that disease. The dermatologist, however, needs to exercise a new kind of suspicion—suspicion of the drug reaction, because it is the drug reaction which has superseded the former specter, syphilis. The drug reaction has become the "Great Imitator."

Tranquilizers offer no substitute for accurate diagnosis or adequate medical supervision. They are adjuncts, likely to displace, but not to replace, some of the older therapies. Physicians who prescribe ataractic drugs indiscriminately are at fault, rather than the drugs themselves.

I have gathered the data contained upon these pages from a search of the medical literature, and my own experience, and I present this monograph with the hope that it may prove helpful to physicians—everywhere.

A. L. W.

ACKNOWLEDGMENT

The author wishes to express his gratitude to Mitchell Ede, M.D., for aid in the preparation of this book. Without his enthusiasm, his cooperation, his diligence, and his learning, completion of this manuscript would not have been possible.

CONTENTS

Section I

The Phenothiazines

PSYCHOTHERAPEUTIC DRUGS

THE PHENOTHIAZINES

Chlorpromazine hydrochloride

Promazine hydrochloride

Triflupromazine hydrochloride

Mepazine

Prochlorperazine

Perphenazine

Trimeprazine

Thorazine hydrochloride

Sparine

Vesprin

Pacatal

Compazine

Trilafon

Temaril

THE PHENOTHIAZINES

INTRODUCTION

The history of the phenothiazine derivatives dates back to 1883 when Bernthsen,[34] while investigating alternate procedures for synthesizing methylene blue, prepared phenothiazine. From that common origin, further study of phenothiazine compounds followed divergent paths. Phenothiazine itself was employed, clinically, as a urinary antiseptic and anthelmintic, but during that employment it was discovered that toxic activities of the drug would preclude its wide application in medicine (with resultant restriction to use in veterinary medicine). In 1945, French investigators began to screen the amine derivatives of phenothiazine, and the over-all results obtained with promethazine (Phenergan) led them to further search for compounds with more marked depressant action on the central nervous system.[134, 272] Meanwhile, German investigators engaged in the synthesis of a number of aromatic (ring) derivatives of phenothiazine. Late in 1950, Charpentier synthesized chlorpromazine,[51, 257] which was introduced in Europe, in 1951, as Largactil, for use in pre-surgery medication. In 1953, Schuler and Nezel (according to Nieschulz and others[169, 170]) reported that mepazine (Pacatal) possessed potential clinical usefulness.

Inasmuch as chlorpromazine hydrochloride (Thorazine Hydrochloride) can be considered the prototype of the phenothiazine compounds, it is with a description of that psychotherapeutic agent that this monograph begins.

CHLORPROMAZINE HYDROCHLORIDE U.S.P.
(*Thorazine Hydrochloride*—Smith Kline & French Laboratories)

Chlorpromazine hydrochloride is 2-chloro-10-(3-dimethylaminopropyl) phenothiazine hydrochloride, which is represented by the following structural formula:

3

Pharmacologic Actions

The unique pharmacologic action of chlorpromazine hydrochloride is a selective inhibition of subcortical centers of the central nervous system—the reticular system of the brain, the thalamus, the hypothalamus, and the autonomic nervous system, without significant action on the cortex, although alertness and spontaneity are reduced.[166] It is believed that the drug acts principally on the higher neural centers in the general area of the diencephalon, selectively inhibiting the chemo-receptor trigger zone (the hypothalamus, and the reticular substance). These centers are believed to control vomiting, heat regulation, wakefulness, vasomotor tone, muscle tone, and secretion from the anterior lobe of the pituitary. Consequently, inhibition of activity in this region affects many psychic and physiological processes, integrated with the central and autonomic nervous systems, and the endocrine systems. While therapeutic results may be due to effects on any one, or a combination of anatomic areas, it is entirely possible that chemical alterations of cerebral metabolic processes rather than anatomic sites of action are responsible for the clinical results obtained with this drug.[276]

Chlorpromazine hydrochloride produces, then, depression of the central nervous system. (Generally, the electroencephalographic patterns are not altered with the usual dose in normal patients, although some variation has occasionally been reported.[23]) Chlorpromazine suppresses or abolishes conditioned reflexes in trained rats. It also exhibits a depressant action on certain neural centers in experimental animals, resulting in suppression of vomiting from apomorphine hydrochloride, irradiation and motion sickness; but the drug does not affect the emesis from morphine, veratrum alkaloids, digitalis and copper sulfate.[125, 166] In addition to these main pharmacological actions, chlorpromazine hydrochloride possesses weak adrenolytic, hypotensive, antispasmodic, hypothermic and antihistaminic effects, and is capable of potentiating the action of many other pharmacological agents.[166]

Administration and Dosage

Chlorpromazine hydrochloride is administered orally, intramuscularly or intravenously. The dosage must be highly individualized, according to the severity of the condition and the degree of response; the smallest effective dose should always be used. Oral dosages range from 10 to 500 mg. or more per day. Dosage for children is reduced, proportionately. Deep intramuscular injection is the preferred parenteral route with the dosage for adults ranging from 25 mg. per day, for mild nausea and vomiting, to as much as 400 mg. per day for acutely agitated manic patients. Because of the added danger of severe hypotension, extreme caution must be exercised in giving the drug intravenously.[166]

Onset of action is rapid, particularly after parenteral administration. Little is known concerning the metabolic fate of the drug in the body,[133] although current evidence suggests the liver as possible site of detoxication. After repeated administration, a slight amount of tolerance develops, particularly to the hypotensive and hypnotic effects.[166]

General Clinical Uses

Chlorpromazine hydrochloride has been found useful for the treatment of the nausea and vomiting associated with certain disorders including carcinomatosis, uremia, acute infections and nitrogen-mustard therapy. Although the use of chlorpromazine hydrochloride in pregnancy for the usual "morning sickness" of the first trimester must be regarded as experimental, it may be tried for controlling hyperemesis gravidarum as a complication of pregnancy, preferably before the onset of liver damage.[166] Its antiemetic effect has been reported as useful in radiation sickness, in the nausea and vomiting produced by certain drugs (including some antibiotics) and for the control of postanesthetic and post-operative nausea and vomiting. It has not been successful in motion sickness.[166]

Chlorpromazine hydrochloride, often, is successful in controlling hiccups, refractory to other forms of therapy, and in the treatment of status asthmaticus.[166] The drug finds its widest use in alleviating manifestations of anxiety, tension, agitation, and in lessening motor activity in both psychoneurotics and psychotics. The latter include selected cases of schizophrenia, mania and toxic and senile psychoses.[6, 7, 17, 130, 149] The sedative, psychotherapeutic and calming properties of the drug also make it useful as an adjunct in the treatment of certain other mental disorders, and in a variety of apparently unrelated conditions where emotional stress is a complicating, or even a causative factor.[149, 237, 259] It has been used successfully in some depressions, in which agitation and anxiety are complications. It appears to be of no value in reducing the frequency or intensity of seizures in epilepsy.[166]

The sedative and antiemetic actions of the drug have been reported to facilitate treatment in acute alcoholism.[240] Its value in narcotic drug withdrawal is not yet established.[166] It has been used in surgical procedures, obstetrics, and in the treatment of severe pain. Its alleged potentiation of hypnotics, sedatives, analgesics and anesthetics is difficult to evaluate.[166] Use of the drug is contraindicated in all comatose patients, or those under the influence of large doses of alcohol, or other central nervous system depressants.[166]

Specific Dermatological Uses

Chlorpromazine hydrochloride has been found to be of adjunctive value in the treatment of certain dermatological conditions, particularly in those cases refractory to other forms of treatment. By no means is the drug a dermatologic panacea; its value lies in its tranquilizing effect. Therefore, the dermatological patient, who responds favorably to chlorpromazine, has some strong emotional factor as a cause of dermatitis, or as a result of dermatitis (such as pruritus and disfigurement). The effectiveness of the drug has been noted in cases of psoriasis,[92] atopic eczema,[37] and neurodermatitis,[236] and in cases of severe pruritis from other causes, where specific therapies have failed.[165, 224] For maximum benefit in the treatment of such conditions, it is necessary to maintain adequate dosage levels for a sufficient period of time. Cornbleet and Barsky[60] have stated:

"It is fruitless to administer small doses of ('Thorazine') for a few days, or a few high doses only. Results are usually observed only after persistent administration, sometimes with gradually increasing dosages, although quite a few cases will show good to excellent response in two to four days after the start of therapy. It is wise to continue medication for some time after good results are obtained because there are significant percentages of relapses. The full benefit of the unique calming effect of 'Thorazine' can be obtained only if the dosage levels are determined individually for each patient."

After the lesions and/or pruritus have subsided, dosage may gradually be reduced to a maintenance level. Should the conditions return, the dosage should be increased.

Chlorpromazine hydrochloride has been found useful in certain cases of intermittent acute porphyria,[159, 161, 233, 247] for the relief of pain and nervousness during acute attacks. No definite evidence has been obtained, at this writing, that a reduced excretion of porphyrins or porphobilinogen may be expected, but it is possible that the drug interrupts a vicious cycle, permitting a spontaneous remission to occur.

A suggested dosage schedule for adults with usual dermatological conditions is shown, following. Dosage for children are proportionately less.[224]

Orally: Start with 25 mg. twice to four times daily. If pruritus is not markedly decreased within 24-48 hours, dosage should be increased by increments of 25 mg. to 50 mg. daily, at semiweekly intervals. Once the optimum dosage level has been established, Thorazine 'Spansules' may be given every 12 hours for sustained 24-hour protection against emotional stress. Usually, not more than 200 mg. daily will be required for control of symptoms.

Intramuscularly: For the rapid control of acute symptoms, 25 mg. (1 cc.) Ampul Solution should be administered intramuscularly with the patient lying down and remaining so, for at least 30 minutes after injection. If necessary, the initial intramuscular dose may be repeated after one hour, if no hypotensive effects occur. Subsequent injections, administered every four to six hours, should be increased until symptoms are controlled. Usually, not more than 50 mg. to 100 mg. three times daily will be required. When symptoms have subsided, and the patient is comfortable and calm, it is usually possible to substitute oral therapy, in amounts equaling previous intramuscular dosage. Local irritation and pain at sites of injections are not unusual.[149]

Because of reported instances of fatal shock, all forms of parenteral administration should, usually, be reserved for bedfast or hospitalized patients.[166]

When necessary, pressor agents, such as phenylephrine hydrochloride or levarterenol bitartrate may be used. Epinephrine should never be chosen for this purpose, since the adrenolytic action of chlorpromazine may cause epinephrine reversal.[166]

Chlorpromazine hydrochloride is a potent agent with complex pharmacological activities. Although its therapeutic range of effectiveness is wide, sufficient experience has not been gained to determine its ultimate place in the therapeutic armamentarium. Physicians, accordingly, should weigh possible beneficial effects against possible toxic reactions and side effects, before prescribing the therapeutic agent.[166]

Toxic Effects and Side Reactions

Dermal Reactions

Margolis and his associates,[156] in 1955, reported nonrecurring chlorpromazine dermatitis. In a series of 53 patients, treated for various psychiatric disorders, seven developed dermatitis of a maculopapular, erythematous, pruritic character. This eruption involved trunk and extremities, but spared face, mucous membranes, palms and soles. It was generalized at onset in five cases, and in two subjects it appeared over a localized area, before becoming diffuse. Time of onset was between the ninth and 37th days of therapy. In six cases, cessation of therapy resulted in disappearance of the eruption within two to seven days. In the seventh subject, the dermatitis cleared over a period of 12 days, without interruption of therapy. In four of these cases, chlorpromazine therapy was resumed shortly after subsidence of the eruption. Medication was started at the 10 mg. oral test dose, and eventually reached dosage levels approximately, and in one case exceeded the dose in force at the time of appearance of the eruption. In two cases not requiring further therapy, no skin reaction occurred after a single 10 mg. oral dose. In one case, it was demonstrated that the eruption cleared without interruption of therapy, or significant reduction in dosage.

Many patients demonstrated increased sensitivity to sunlight. Fourteen developed erythema on repeated occasions, after relatively mild exposure, and two developed a fine vesicular eruption, after moderate exposure.

Mullins and his associates,[165] in 1956, reported various cutaneous sensitivity reactions to chlorpromazine hydrochloride.

"Our series consists of 85 patients manifesting skin eruptions due to chlorpromazine. It does not include approximately 200 other patients who have been observed but on whom records were inadequate for purposes of this study. Fifty-seven patients presented some type of generalized reaction."

This group was subdivided according to the following types of cutaneous eruptions:

erythematous morbilliform with edema
urticarious
seborrheic
purpuric
papular
bullous
miliaria-like

Although there were purpuric and petechial eruptions, in some instances, there were no alterations of platelet counts.

Total daily dosage, which ranged from 50 mg. to 1.2 Gm., played little part in the production of photosensitization reactions. Most of the eruptions in this category were of the papulovesicular variety and occurred at the sites of exposure. One severe bullous eruption appeared within two hours after a 20-minutes' exposure to sunshine. The lesions produced by photosensitization, with the exception of the single bullous reaction, were deep-seated, indicating that the site of disturbance was probably in the upper cutis. A considerable degree of brawny-type edema was associated with these lesions.

During hot summer months, many patients demonstrated a sweat-gland obstructive reaction in the form of a miliaria-like eruption—the majority being of the miliaria-crystallina type. Some of these cases, however, seemed to have deeper obstruction of the sweat pores.

In several cases, individuals predisposed to seborrhea had a decided flare of their seborrheic dermatitis.

Ten cases of contact dermatitis were observed.

As can be seen, chlorpromazine can, and does produce almost every type of cutaneous eruption. It is interesting to note that no mucous membrane lesions were observed.

Patch testing of patients, as well as several hundred volunteers, revealed that "this substance is a primary irritant when applied at full strength. This suggests that patch tests are of little value in determining whether a patient might react to chlorpromazine given systemically."

Many features about reactions to chlorpromazine are a decided variation from reactions to other systemically administered medicaments. First, there is produced a minimal amount of symptomatology, as compared with other drug reactions. Second, eruptions clear quite rapidly, in a period of two to five days after therapy is discontinued. Once the dosage has been decreased or discontinued, lesions disappear, and, in the majority of cases studied, chlorpromazine can be re-administered without recurrence of the eruption.

Nonrecurring athrombocytopenic purpura has been reported by Shannon, et al.[219]

*

Urticaria has been mentioned by a number of investigators.[55, 129, 165, 274] Raymer[190] has remarked that urticarial lesions caused by oral administration of chlorpromazine, in one case, were of a fixed-type, rather than the usual migratory eruption, ordinarily expected in urticaria.

*

Lewis and Sawicky[145] were the first to sound the alarm regarding contact dermatitis:

"In spite of attempts by the pharmaceutical firm to predict an incidence of contact sensitivity, the work failed to reveal the danger to those who handle chlorpromazine frequently or over a prolonged period. Since this problem concerns chiefly nurses or physicians, it is of added importance to the profession that the possibility of severe epidermal sensitization to chlorpromazine be appreciated. Failure to recognize promptly the causal agent and to institute suitable measures to prevent contact with the drug will subject the patient to the hazard of an incapacitating dermatitis."

These investigators reported two cases, both in nurses exposed to the drug frequently, and over prolonged periods, indicating that individuals become sensitized to chlorpromazine. In both cases, the resulting dermatitis was sufficiently severe to be entirely disabling; the course, unusually protracted.

Contact dermatitis has been reported by others.[149, 217, 249, 274]

Hospital nurses, who have become sensitized to chlorpromazine, upon return to work wearing masks and gloves, and using every other precaution, have been known to have recurrence of generalized dermatitis requiring hospitalization, after being exposed only to fumes from broken vials of the drug.[46]

A dentist working on psychotic patients, under therapy with chlorpromazine hydrochloride, has been known to develop dermatitis on the fingers which contacted the patients' saliva.[58]

*

Cahn and Levy[42] reported, in the American literature, that in some chlorpromazine-treated patients, puritic, erythematopapular eruptions appeared on parts of the body exposed to intense summer sunlight. Usually, pruritus subsided within two hours after the patient took cover—and the eruption disappeared within 24 hours.

"These lesions apparently are precipitated by ultraviolet rays of 2,968 to 3,025 A° in length, which are present in summer, but not in winter sunlight. This hypothesis is substantiated by the observation that exposure to ultraviolet light from a hot quartz mercury arc lamp, which emits a scattered spectrum unlike the continuous spectrum of summer sunlight, produces erythema with equal rapidity in patients who have had chlorpromazine dermatitis, patients who have had no side effects from chlorpromazine therapy, and persons who are not receiving the drug.

"Since the skin reaction is transitory, photosensitivity does not necessitate withdrawal of chlorpromazine. However, the patients should be warned to avoid overexposure to summer sunlight."

The conclusions of Cahn and Levy were supported by the

findings of John A. Epstein, and his co-workers.[74] The mechanism for the abnormal reaction to sun induced by chlorpromazine, according to these investigators, remains obscure. Ultraviolet rays with wave lengths shorter than 3,100 A° are not likely to be involved in photodynamic reactions. However, since the absorption spectrum of chlorpromazine includes such rays, the drug may act as a light-absorber for some photochemical reaction (probably not photodynamic in nature). This would require permeation of the drug into the epidermis. On the other hand, chlorpromazine, or its transformation products might act directly on epidermal cells. Still another possible mechanism of this exaggerated sunburn reaction may be related to the potent effects of the drug upon blood vessels. Chlorpromazine appears to cause vasodilatation through central and peripheral actions. Since the erythema noted in the normal sunburn response is due to dilatation of the dermal blood vessels, a substance which would tend to enhance this vasodilatation might conceivably cause an exaggerated response. Finally, the possibility of a photoallergic process, also, must be considered.

Clinical and experimental investigations on photodynamic effects of phenothiazine derivatives, particularly of chlorpromazine, were reported in the European literature by Schulz, Wiskemann and Wulf,[209] who demonstrated several categories of sensitivity, summarized following:

a phototoxic reaction based on the photodynamic action, which occurred in all the subjects, who were tested;

a photoallergic reaction in which the patch test with the drug alone was negative, but which could be demonstrated by irradiation of the patch test site;

a photoallergic reaction in combination with an allergic eczematous contact-type sensitization, in which the patch test was positive with the phenothiazine derivative alone, but a stronger response was elicited if the patch test site were irradiated.

Following publication of these European studies, Stephan Epstein and Rowe[75] reported a case of photosensitivity to promethazine (Phenergan) and chlorpromazine. Originally, contact sensitivity could be demonstrated only to Phenergan; but photocross-sensitivity existed, at the same time, also, to chlorpromazine. The allergen, they concluded, in this photoallergic reaction was different from the original drug, probably an oxidation or decomposition product.

Stephan Epstein has reported, also, on photosensitization dermatitis following application of Phenergan, and photosensitization dermatitis due to systemically-administered Phenergan.[19]

Photosensitivity, as a side effect of chlorpromazine therapy, has been reported by other investigators.[274]

*

Space does not permit detailed discussion of all the side effects of chlorpromazine therapy, but the following pages will provide itemization of those manifestations of toxic effects and side reactions.

Allergic Phenomena

Edema, periorbital, facial, pretibial, pedal......7, 99, 149, 259, 269
Edema, laryngeal, requiring immediate hospitalization in a
    patient who had had a previous reaction to penicillin......39
Eosinophilia......149, 152, 232, 269
Influenza-like syndrome with fever, generalized weakness,
    myalgia, arthralgia......129, 149
Nasal congestion, without rhinorrhea......99, 259, 269, 274
Toxic liver changes......6, 7, 17, 36, 55, 99, 115, 117, 126, 129, 135,
                140, 149, 152, 162, 175, 202, 228, 232, 235,
                237, 241, 258, 269

1. Obstructive-type jaundice without indication of previous liver dysfunction, occurring during therapy, or after its discontinuance, without relation to dosage, and characterized by symptoms of intermittent nausea, generalized pruritus, urticaria, icterus: or, by fever, elevated phosphatase level and eosinophilia, as the only indications. There is customarily an elevation of the serum alkaline phosphatase and serum cholesterol, with little or no disturbance of the cephalin flocculation and thymol turbidity. Microscopically, there is stasis of bile in the intralobular canaliculi, with or without inflammatory infiltration.

Wound-bleeding, in chlorpromazine-jaundiced patients, is not explainable on the basis of hypoprothrombinemia, coagulation defect, abnormal bleeding time, or capillary fragility 152

Cardiovascular Complications

Central Nervous System Effects

Ocular manifestations—
Blurred vision_____232, 269
Miosis _____232, 269
Mydriasis _____232, 269
Myostatic phenomena_____232
Seizures: convulsions_____23, 107, 109, 149, 157, 203

Endocrine Imbalances

Delay in ovulation and menstruation_____22, 251
Galactorrhea _____22, 129, 270, 274
Impotence _____274
Increased sexual desire _____274
Mammary tissue-growth _____129, 189
Transient hyperglycemia and glycosuria: previously-
controlled diabetes becoming unstabilized_____114

Gastrointestinal Disturbances

Anti-emesis _____8, 20
     When intestinal obstruction is present, symptoms may
be masked, thus delaying intervention to the point of
irreversibility.
     Existence, or course of intra-abdominal malignancy
may be masked_____8
Constipation _____6, 149, 274
Decrease in gastric secretion:
indigestion and pyrosis_____6, 8, 232, 269, 274
Nausea _____129, 149
Voracious appetite and weight gain_____149, 269, 274
     Increased appetite and fluid intake may precipitate
frequency of micturition_____149

Hematopoietic Changes

Blood dyscrasias _____36, 166
     Chlorpromazine "should be immediately discontinued
if patients exhibit evidence of bone marrow depression:
physicians should also be alert for any toxic hematopoietic
effects, fever or sore throat."
Agranulocytosis _____6, 8, 36, 44, 115, 118, 148,
                                          149, 198, 202, 204, 235

The Robinsons[278] have reported study of 2,087 patients with various dermatoses aggravated by psychogenic factors, to whom were administered, for periods varying from eight weeks to two years, various drugs for the control of emotional tension. Ataractic drugs were administered to 637 of these patients. One of the ataractic drugs, chlorpromazine, was administered to 100 patients, in individualized dosages ranging from 5 mg. to 1,000 mg. three or four times daily. Subjective relief was afforded by the drug to 80% of that series. There were no serious side effects or reactions. The conclusion of these investigators was:

"Thorazine has limited usefulness in the field of dermatology."

The author and his associate have observed response to chlorpromazine by a slightly smaller series, 87 patients, to whom the drug was administered in individualized dosages ranging from 5 mg. to 500 mg. three or four times daily, during intervals ranging from six weeks to 18 months. All patients had emotional factors complicating or aggravating their dermatoses.

Sainz[202] has reported:

"Over 50% of patients treated with chlorpromazine show some associated side reaction."

In our series, 48 of 87 patients exhibited associated toxic effects and side reactions, and while none was serious, it is our wish to confirm the conclusion of the Robinsons: chlorpromazine does, indeed, have limited usefulness in dermatological practice.

PROMAZINE HYDROCHLORIDE N.N.D.
(*Sparine*—Wyeth Laboratories)

Promazine hydrochloride is 10-(3-dimethylaminopropyl)-phenothiazine hydrochloride.

The compound is identical with chlorpromazine hydrochloride, except that it lacks the chlorine atom on the ring structure, as can be seen from the following formula.

Promazine Hydrochloride   Chlorpromazine Hydrochloride

Pharmacologic Actions

The general pharmacological properties of these two pheno-thiazine derivatives are likewise very similar, the chief difference being a lower acute toxicity with promazine, after oral and paren-teral administration to experimental animals. Milligram for milli-gram, in laboratory and clinical investigations, promazine hydro-chloride has been shown to be one-third to one-fourth as potent as chlorpromazine in its pharmacologic actions (e.g., adrenolytic and depressant properties) yet in equivalent therapeutic doses, the inci-dence of seizures and toxic confusional states has been greater with promazine, than with chlorpromazine.[166, 274]

Certain investigators[11, 276] have shown that the principal site of action of the promazines appears to be in the upper brain stem, where possibly these drugs interfere, in some way, with utilization of adenosine triphosphate.

Administration and Dosage

The amount, route of administration and frequency of dose of promazine hydrochloride should be governed by the severity of the condition treated, and the response of the patient. For maximum therapeutic benefit, dosages must be individualized for each patient. The oral route of administration should be used whenever possible, but when nausea, vomiting or lack of cooperation is evident, promazine may be given intravenously or intramuscularly. In general, parenteral administration should be reserved for bedfast patients, although acute states in ambulatory patients may be treated by injection, provided proper precautions are taken to eliminate the possibility of postural hypotension.[166] Promazine hydrochloride is tolerated by either intravenous or intramuscular administration, and while its use is not attended by any degree of local discomfort or irritation,[79] care must be exercised not to allow perivascular extravasation, since under such circumstances, chemical irritation may be severe.

In the management of agitated patients, it is recommended that promazine may be given intravenously in initial doses of 50 to 150 mg. If the desired calming effect is not apparent within five to ten minutes, additional doses up to a total of 300 mg. may be given. Once the desired effect is obtained, the drug may be administered intramuscularly, or orally. The oral or intramuscular dose is 10 mg. to 200 mg., at intervals of four to six hours.

In less severe disturbances, the oral route may be satisfactory for initiating therapy. Maintenance dosage may range from 10 to 200 mg., given at intervals of four to six hours. When tablet medication is unsuitable, or refused, Sparine Syrup, or Sparine Liquid Concentrate may be used by diluting in appropriate citrus or chocolate-flavored drinks.

It is recommended that the total daily dose of promazine hydrochloride not exceed 1,000 mg. For children, dosages are proportionately less.

General Clinical Uses

Promazine hydrochloride is used in the same manner as chlorpromazine hydrochloride, for the treatment of acute neuropsychiatric agitation.[7,17,25,79,90,160,185,239] The drug effectively allays apprehension and anxiety, which accompany various types of acute psychoses; it is also reported to be useful in the management of such alcohol-induced syndromes as delirium-tremens, acute hallucinosis and tremulousness.

First-reported results from use of promazine hydrochloride for the treatment of psychotic patients were more satisfactory than results obtained in similar groups, treated with chlorpromazine.[79,160] No serious side effects were encountered. Late in 1956, however, Woodward and Solomon[256] described a case of fatal agranulycytosis, occurring in a patient on the 48th day of promazine hydrochloride administration (dosage having been instituted at 100 mg. daily, reaching a maximum of 1 Gm., in four divided doses), over a 42-day period.

In October of 1957, there appeared this Report (of the Council) on blood dyscrasias associated with promazine hydrochloride therapy:[35]

"A review of the reports received by the Registry since July, 1956, revealed 10 cases of blood dyscrasias apparently associated with promazine (Sparine) hydrochloride therapy. A search of the English language medical literature to date of the preparation of this statement has uncovered two case reports of granulocytopenia associated with promazine hydrochloride therapy, one of which is among those reported to the Registry. Wyeth Laboratories has been most cooperative and has supplied an additional record of 8 cases not previously reported to the Registry, bringing the total to 18 cases in which promazine therapy was suspected as being associated with a case of blood dyscrasia."

Further:

"Although depression of granulocytes was prominent in every case reported, the bone marrow studies in some cases indicated a depression of other cellular elements as well. Of the 18 known cases, we have information that 4 ended fatally."

Finally:

"Since the drug may possess potential for some harm, the subcommittee suggests that physicians limit its use to those conditions in which such use is warranted and avoid its use in the treatment of trivial or minor complaints."

Specific Dermatological Uses

Therapy with promazine hydrochloride in dermatological conditions has not, to the author's knowledge, been undertaken. However, that dermatologists do encounter patients on therapy with this drug, is illustrated by the following:

For a female patient with atopic eczema, aged 19 years, under the author's care and continuous dermatological supervision for the past ten years, promazine hydrochloride, in a total daily dosage of 750 mg., was prescribed by a family physician, who made no effort to obtain information on the patient's past or present internal therapeutic regimens. Prescription of the drug was justified (in his opinion) inasmuch as the patient had complained of "jitteriness" and "nervousness."

A consultation between general practitioner and dermatologist resulted in agreement that for the promazine hydrochloride, there might be substituted some other medication, equally effective for nervous tension—a medicament which was known to possess no high "potential for harm." (Incidentally, the patient had taken promazine hydrochloride for three weeks, before she reported for her regular monthly dermatological re-check. Hemogram showed slight alteration, which was reversed within a month after cessation of therapy.)

The above is cited to illustrate the contention that physicians, who prescribe psychotherapeutic agents, indiscriminately, are at fault—rather than the drugs themselves.

Toxic Effects and Side Reactions

In view of the close structural relationship, it is possible that any of the untoward reactions attributed to chlorpromazine could occur, following administration of promazine hydrochloride.

Dermal Reactions

In an early study on the use of promazine hydrochloride in psychiatric patients, Usdin[239] reported that in a series of 30 patients, urticaria, or generalized rash appeared in two subjects—one patient developing urticaria after five doses of 25 mg. each. The eruption subsided upon discontinuance of the drug, and administration of an antihistamine. There have been other observations of cutaneous eruptions,[11,17,185] in some instances severe enough to warrant cessation of therapy.

Atkinson[11] reported, in his clinical experience with promazine hydrochloride in the treatment of psychiatric patients, one case of severe glossitis, which he listed as a side effect of therapy.

Allergic Phenomena

Edema[17] has been observed. Jaundice has not been reported; however, Kinross-Wright[274] observed an instance of severe right upper quadrant pain, nausea and vomiting, associated with an elevated serum alkaline phosphatase. He considered these symptoms to be highly suggestive of the chlorpromazine-type of hepatic involvement.

Cardiovascular Complications

Hypotension, dizziness, syncope and tachycardia have been reported.[11,17,79,160,185] There have been instances of vasomotor, or impending collapse,[11,17] with systolic blood pressure falling below 60 mm./hg., accompanied by shock-like syndrome. Fatality with this syndrome has been reported.[274]

Central Nervous System Effects

Photophobia occurred in two patients observed by Usdin.[239] This side effect of therapy appeared during the first two to four days of medication, disappeared without treatment, and did not recur when the drug was continued for six weeks in one case, and seven weeks, in the other. Prescod and Townley[185] observed photophobia, which they attributed to the atropine-like action of promazine hydrochloride.

The following have been reported by a number of investigators:

Convulsions: seizures_____17, 25, 137, 243
    Fazekas et al. observed that phenothiazine derivatives
    have a capacity, in large doses administered to susceptible
    patients, to precipitate seizures _____266
    Kinross-Wright has likewise remarked on the capacity
    of promazine to precipitate seizures_____274
Depersonalization _____11
Depression _____239
Dreams: nightmares_____11
Drowsiness: somnolence_____11, 160, 185, 239, 274
Hyperthermia _____17
Lethargy _____160, 239
Xerostomia _____11, 185, 274

Gastrointestinal Disturbances

Hematopoietic Changes

TRIFLUPROMAZINE HYDROCHLORIDE
(*Vesprin*—E. R. Squibb & Sons)

Triflupromazine hydrochloride is 10-(3-dimethylamino-pro-pyl)-2-(trifluoromethyl) phenothiazine hydrochloride, a compound having in its chemical structure an amino side-chain (as does chlorpromazine), wherein fluorine has been substituted for chlorine. The structural formula for this compound is shown, following:

$$CH_2\text{-}CH_2\text{-}CH_2\text{-}N(CH_3)_2\text{-}HCl$$

Kinross-Wright pointed out that substitution of fluorine for chlorine in the chemical structure was accomplished in an effort to reduce autonomic effects: that such substitution served to increase potency, weight for weight.[270]

Pharmacologic Actions

In laboratory animals, the effects of triflupromazine hydrochloride have been found to be similar to those of chlorpromazine, and in certain respects, more potent.[16, 179] Triflupromazine has depressant and sedative effects in mice. Its tranquilizing influence in monkeys is five times more potent than that of chlorpromazine; and almost three times more potent in inhibiting conditioned reflex responses in rats. Triflupromazine has some morphine-potentiating and anti-LSD pyretogenic effects. It has a milder hypotensive effect than chlorpromazine, and perhaps less activity on vegetative nervous systems. It possesses moderate anti-histaminic activity, and like chlorpromazine inhibits Pitocin, serotonin and spontaneous uterine activity of guinea-pigs.

A comparison of the cardiovascular dynamics of triflupromazine with chlorpromazine has demonstrated[91] that the immediate effect of both drugs on blood pressure was about equal, but there was less profound depression of the arterial pressure with triflupromazine. The immediate effect on the heart rate, following administration of triflupromazine, was a transient rise, followed by a rapid fall to slightly below normal, as a persistent effect. Both drugs depressed the carotid pressor reflex, and partially inhibited the tachycardic responses to acetylcholines. Generally, triflupromazine was less active in the latter responses than chlorpromazine.

Administration and Dosage

Triflupromazine may be administered orally: 25 mg. three times daily, initially, with adjustment of dosage according to patient response, and with caution in daily doses of 300 mg.; and intramuscularly, 1 cc. (20 mg./cc.) of Parenteral Solution, three times daily, with caution in exceeding doses of 150 mg. The intramuscular administration of the drug has been found to be much less irritating than intramuscular administration of chlorpromazine "particularly since somewhat less medication is required and the solution is somewhat less acid."[102]

General Clinical Uses

Triflupromazine is a potent behavior-modifier, intended for the management of the seriously agitated and disturbed patient. Clinical appraisal has demonstrated that the drug is at least twice as potent in controlling psychotic manifestations as chlorpromazine. It is useful in the management of psychomotor agitation associated with various acute and chronic psychoses including schizophrenia, mania, depression, delirium, senile psychoses, psychoses due to organic brain damage. It is useful in the management of the alcohol-withdrawal syndrome.

Specific Dermatological Uses

Treatment of dermatological patients with triflupromazine has not, to the author's knowledge, been undertaken. However, study has been made of the effect of the drug in inducing photosensitivity in humans.[43] In the test-group, consisting of 70 normal male volunteers, there was one significant reaction, which is here summarized. The patient, a normal white male, aged 36 years, was exposed to both Hanovia Hot Quartz light and Therapeutic "C" carbon arc high-intensity burner, and normal reactions were recorded. The patient then ingested 25 mg. triflupromazine three times daily for one month, and was re-exposed to irradiation. An intense erythema developed at the site of the carbon arc exposure (4 + erythema) starting at 10-second exposure (normally one erythema dose in this subject). No difference was observed to the Hanovia Hot Quartz light exposures, before therapy, or following it.

The investigators concluded, on the basis of this experiment, that the patient was sensitive to ultraviolet rays between 2967 and 3025 A°, presumably due to triflupromazine.

" . . . it must be assumed that Vesprin is capable of causing photosensitivity in human subjects in a very small percentage of cases.

Such photosensitivity would only occur due to a very narrow wave band, 2967-3025 A°, present only in summer sunlight, and of great intensity. Hence, patients taking the drug would not develop photosensitivity except under these exacting situations of exposure."

In a clinical trial of triflupromazine, administered to patients with mental syndromes, Azima[16] reported that one patient became markedly photosensitive following Vesprin therapy. (There were 39 patients in his series, under therapy for an interval of two to three weeks, on dosages of triflupromazine ranging from 50 mg. to 400 mg. daily, with the average dose, 200 mg.). According to Azima:

"This sensitivity was much greater than with chlorpromazine, which was administered subsequently instead of Vesprin, because the patient could not tolerate the least amount of sunshine."

Photosensitivity was also manifested by a patient in a study of Vesprin, reported by Goldman.[102]

Toxic Effects and Side Reactions

Dermal Reactions

In Goldman's series of 177 patients, toxic effects and side reactions were manifested in 62 individuals. He found:

"The dermatologic manifestations of triflupromazine are characteristically of allergic type and similar to those produced by chlorpromazine."

He observed development of "rash" in three patients, and conjunctivitis, in two patients.

Freed[95] reported the interesting case of a 40-year old female who was put on triflupromazine therapy because of a severe character neurosis. She had previously developed an urticarial type of skin reaction to chlorpromazine, with large wheals on her face and arms; but a different type of dermatitis appeared after the patient took Vesprin, 50 mg., three times daily for approximately three weeks. The latter eruption was morbilliform in type; it appeared only on the arms; the local subjective sensations consisted of stinging and burning, rather than itching. Lesions subsided when therapy was stopped. Freed made this comment:

"The fact that the patient had responded differently in abnormal skin reactions to chlorpromazine and Vesprin points up the opportunity afforded to investigate the possibility of specific system reactions to individual drugs."

Gallagher and Pfeiffer[98] observed that two patients with schizophrenia, one male and one female, developed marked oiliness of the skin, while taking Vesprin, for a prolonged interval.

Allergic Phenomena

Edema has been reported:[102] also, edema invloving one hand, and the feet, in the same individual.[16]

Cardiovascular Complications

Bradycardia --91
Hypertension, concomitant with increased anxiety

Hematopoietic Changes

Gallagher and Pfeiffer[98] reported that leukocyte counts tended to decrease, in both male and female groups, observed by them: however, abnormally low counts did not occur. The differential leukocyte counts gave no indication of the occurrence of intoxication.

MEPAZINE
*(Pacatal—*Warner-Chilcott Laboratories)

Mepazine is 10-(N-methyl-3-piperidylmethyl)-phenothiazine, which is represented by the following structural formula:

Pharmacologic Actions

Mepazine has been found to exert, in animal experiments as well as in clinical practice, a selective regulating action upon the central nervous system without inhibiting the cortical centers. The drug produces tranquility, without hypnosis, and although large doses may induce sleep, the patient is nevertheless easily aroused and consciousness remains clear. The sympathetic and parasympathetic systems, both involved in emotional behavior, are inhibited. The drug possesses mild antihistaminic, antipyretic and antispasmodic activity. It has been shown to have vasopressor and vasodilator effects, but weak hypotensive action. Mepazine has exhibited vasodilator effects on the coronary vessels of the isolated guinea-pig heart, and spasmolytic effect upon induced coronary spasm in the rat, this effect being stronger than that exerted by papaverine.

Administration and Dosage

Mepazine may be administered orally, or intramuscularly, in dosages which are individualized for the needs of each patient. The initial dose should be low. For the ambulant patient, an oral dose of 25 mg. three or four times daily is recommended, with gradual increase of 25 mg./day if indicated, every five to seven days, until the patient is controlled, calm and cooperative. The optimal dose should be continued for about two weeks before reducing the amount gradually, to the lowest possible maintenance level. Oral dosages for hospitalized patients may be higher. The severely agitated patient may receive the drug by intramuscular injection, 50 mg. (2 cc. Ampul Solution) three or four times daily. Injections must be given deeply and slowly. Pain and local irritation may be particularly noticeable when large doses of the drug are administered.[64] If hypotension occurs, ephedrine can be injected intravenously, to restore blood pressure to normal.

General Clinical Uses

Mepazine has been found clinically effective in the treatment of manic states; schizophrenia; involutional psychoses; excessive psychomotor activity;[81] paranoid psychoses; obsessive-compulsive neuroses; anxiety neuroses; senile dementia; drug withdrawal syndrome; and chronic alcoholism.[82] The drug has been found useful for potentiation of analgesics and narcotics in advanced carcinoma; and during labor.[188] In anesthesia and surgery, mepazine has appeared to reduce, in certain cases, preoperative tension and anxiety, and to provide a smooth induction phase.[64] As with chlorpromazine, however, mepazine is contraindicated for patients in coma, under the influence of large quantities of alcohol, or other central nervous system depressants. In certain cases of epilepsy, mepazine has apparently potentiated the sedative effects of anticonvulsant drugs.[101]

Mepazine must be administered with great care to patients with a history of jaundice, liver damage, or drug sensitivity.

Specific Dermatological Uses

Study of mepazine in dermatological patients was undertaken by the author and his associate (with the realization that such potent phrenotropic agent could have but limited application in dermatological therapy). For our study, all patients were drawn from private practice; all were observed at weekly intervals; and only those who faithfully followed prescribed therapeutic regimens were included in evaluation of results.

Mepazine was the sole internal therapeutic agent administered for tranquilizing effect. Topical therapeutic regimens were varied as conditions required, and in some cases there was concomitant administration of actinic therapy. The history of each patient was subjected to critical scrutiny before institution of therapy, so that patients with any indication of liver dysfunction or predisposition to seizures were eliminated. Pertinent data, such as normal hemograms, urinalyses, blood pressures and pulse rates were recorded for comparative purposes.

Our study included

32 females............ranging in age from 22-54 years
10 males ....ranging in age from 26-59 years

All patients had dermatoses complicated by known psychogenic factors. Diagnoses of these patients are shown, following:

	Females	Males
Allergic conjunctivitis	1	--
Atopic dermatitis	6	--
Chronic infectious eczematoid dermatitis	8	4
Contact dermatitis	5	1
Erythema multiforme	--	1
Neurodermatitis	2	--
Pruritus ani et vulvae	3	2
Psoriasis	4	1
Seborrheic dermatitis	3	1
Totals	32	10

The initial dosage schedule was mepazine 25 mg. twice or thrice daily, after meals, or after certain meals and at bedtime. In a few patients, this dosage was reduced to 25 mg. once daily. In only four patients did we observe response to a dosage of 25 mg. four times daily. Urinalyses and hemograms were done on 24 patients, who received the drug for periods ranging from four to six weeks. Sulfobromophthalein (bromsulphalein) test was made on one patient, who received the drug for 12 weeks. All tests were within normal limits.

Our evaluation of response to medication was based on increase or decrease in excoriations and/or erythema; and on subjective improvement, or lack of it, reported by the patient. The following side effects (observed by us, or reported by the patients) were manifested either singly or in combination in a total of 39 patients:

	Females	Males
Drowsiness: hangover	8	6
Dizziness	6	3
"Unable to stand"	1	1
The patients who made this comment said, when they were questioned, they meant they felt "weak."		
Dysphagia	2	--
Difficulties in accommodation	2	1
"Can't see so well—need to have my eyes examined."		
Nausea: anorexia	1	2

Dermatitis --- 1   --

Constipation -- 13   3

One female patient, who consulted us because of allergic conjunctivitis, and who had no manifestations of cutaneous eruption, developed a maculopapular rash on her forearms, during the third week of medication on a dosage schedule of 25 mg. twice daily. When the drug was discontinued, the eruption cleared. One month later, this patient was given mepazine again, in the same dosage (without the patient's knowledge) during an interval of two weeks. The dermatitis did not recur.

Three patients (two females and one male) with generalized seborrheic dermatitis of long-standing, manifested decided flares of their eruptions. Whether or not this was due to the drug, or to other factors, is not known, but it will be recalled that other investigators[165] have observed a similar exacerbation of seborrheic dermatitis in patients, as a result of therapy with chlorpromazine.

In four patients, when a dosage of 25 mg. three times daily did not provide sufficient relief from tension, a dosage of 100 mg. mepazine daily was administered for intervals of two to three weeks. The higher dosage seemed to produce only greater drowsiness and somnolence.

One male psoriatic patient, under our care for eight years, who had at various intervals, tried without relief of pruritus, barbiturates, antihistamines and tranquilizing drugs other than phenothiazine derivatives, not only tolerated mepazine in a dosage of 75 mg. daily, but said he felt better than he had for years. (This patient was on mepazine therapy for 12 weeks.)

Originally, we had planned to use substitution therapy with placebo medication in all patients, but response to therapy did not appear to warrant such use, except in five patients. Substitution of the placebo was made during the fifth week of therapy, and without the patient's knowledge. At the end of a month, three patients told us that therapy with the placebo was "working just as well as ever," and two patients offered the comment that "the medicine was losing its effect."

We conclude from our observations that mepazine is undoubtedly therapeutically active, but use in dermatological patients (particularly ambulatory dermatological patients), is seriously limited by troublesome, if not potentially dangerous side effects. In this conclusion, we confirm the opinion of Ayd.[260]

Toxic Effects and Side Reactions

Dermal Reactions

Dermatitis 93, 260, 271
Photosensitivity 260

Allergic Phenomena

Jaundice 260, 271
Pyrexia 101, 263

Cardiovascular Complications

Hypotension 263, 271

Central Nervous System Effects

Confusion 263
Difficulties in accommodation...263, 271
Dizziness 271
Drowsiness: somnolence 93, 263, 271
Extrapyramidal dysfunction: Toxic paralysis of the powers
    of accommodation, giving rise to visual disturbances,
    bladder atonia, marked constipation, and paralytic ileus
    have been reported..260
    Parkinsonism 263, 271
Seizures: convulsions..260, 271
Xerostomia 93, 101, 260, 263, 271

Endocrine Imbalances

Disturbance of menstruation...81, 82
    (Transient albuminuria may develop, which disappears
when the drug is stopped, and does not recur when the
drug is re-administered, according to report made to
Warner-Chilcott by one of their investigators. See manufacturer's literature.)

Gastrointestinal Disturbances

Anorexia 101, 271
Constipation 101, 260, 271
(See page 31)
Nausea and vomiting 101, 271
Paralytic ileus 260, 271
(See page 31)

According to Gillie, nausea, anorexia, and vomiting have been known to persist in mentally defective children, treated with mepazine, for as long as one or two weeks following cessation of medication.

Hematopoietic Changes

Blood dyscrasias:
Agranulocytosis 271
with fatality 81, 82
Eosinophilia 81, 82
Granulocytopenia 260, 271
Leukopenia 263

PROCHLORPERAZINE
PROCHLORPERAZINE ETHANEDISULFONATE
PROCHLORPERAZINE MALEATE

(*Compazine, Compazine Ethanedisulfonate* and *Compazine Dimaleate*—Smith Kline & French Laboratories)

Prochlorperazine is 2-chloro-10-[3-(1-methyl-4-piperazinyl) propyl] phenothiazine.[184] It has the same actions and uses as prochlorperazine maleate, except that it is administered rectally. Prochlorperazine ethanedisulfonate is 2-chloro-10-[3-(1-methyl-4-piperazinyl) propyl] phenothiazine ethanedisulfonate.[186] It has the same actions and uses as prochlorperazine maleate, except that it may be administered intramuscularly as well as orally. Prochlorperazine maleate is 2-chloro-10-[3-(1-methyl-4-piperazinyl) propyl] phenothiazine dimaleate,[186] which is administered orally. Structural formulae for these three compounds are shown, following:

Prochlorperazine

Prochlorperazine Ethanedisulfonate

Pharmacologic Actions

On a weight basis, prochlorperazine is considerably more potent than chlorpromazine, and comparable therapeutic effects may be achieved with doses which are approximately one-fifth of the latter agent.[186] The drug produces less adrenergic blockade, and consequently less hypotension than does chlorpromazine. Prochlorperazine exerts, also, mild antihistaminic and antispasmodic effects. In experimental animals, prochlorperazine blocks conditioned reflexes, without appreciably affecting motor activity. Unlike chlorpromazine, its potentiating action on other central nervous system depressants is minimal, and may be clinically insignificant. The precise mechanism of action, metabolic fate, and excretion of prochlorperazine are not known.[186]

Administration and Dosage

Prochlorperazine is administered rectally. The usual dosage for adults: one 25 mg. Compazine Suppository twice daily; for children up to two years of age, one-half to one 5 mg. suppository twice daily; two to six years of age, one 5 mg. suppository twice daily; and six to 12 years of age, one or more 5 mg. suppositories twice daily.

Prochlorperazine ethanedisulfonate may be administered intramuscularly: (Ampuls, 2 cc., containing 5 mg./cc. of prochlorperazine as the ethanedisulfonate). Inasmuch as parenteral therapy is usually reserved for the treatment of severe nausea and vomiting, and acute disturbed psychotics, dosage schedules are not included here, but can be found in the manufacturer's literature. Dosage schedule for orally administered ethanedisulfonate is: for adults and children, the same as for the prochlorperazine maleate—the ethanedisulfonate being in syrup form (5 mg./teaspoon) and the maleate in tablet form, or as a sustained-release capsule.

The oral dose of prochlorperazine maleate for adults with mild to moderate emotional disturbances and nausea and vomiting ranges from 5 mg.-10 mg. three or four times daily. For infants and children up to two years of age, 0.25 mg. per pound body weight one or two times daily, but not exceeding a total of 15 mg. daily; for children two to six years of age, 5 mg. two or three times daily, but not exceeding 20 mg. daily; and for children six to 12 years of age, the usual oral dose is 5 mg. two or three times daily, but not exceeding a total of 25 mg. per day.

General Clinical Uses

Prochlorperazine is employed for the treatment of those neuroses and mild emotional disturbances in which anxiety, tension and agitation predominate.[150] The drug is apparently capable of alleviating this type of mental stress, and of lessening motor activity in a sizable percentage of patients.[142] Prochlorperazine has been employed in severe psychiatric disorders, such as schizophrenia, mania, involutional psychoses, degenerative conditions, and senile and toxic psychoses. On the basis of subjective observations, the drug appears to be useful in many such cases. Beneficial results ascribed to its action include, among other things, reduction in psychomotor agitation and excitement, diminished aggressiveness and destructiveness, loss of hallucinations and delusions, and a general calming effect. The drug has been used successfully in some cases of psychomotor retardation marked by apathy and lethargy. Prochlorperazine may be effectively employed as an anti-emetic,[106, 231] and for this purpose exhibits a potency of about four or five times that of chlorpromazine. In general, the over-all clinical toxicity of prochlorperazine appears to be somewhat less than that of chlorpromazine.

Specific Dermatological Uses

The author and his associate have observed response of a small series of 24 patients (drawn from private practice) to prochlorperazine maleate prescribed for the relief of anxiety and tension complicating various dermatoses. The drug was administered orally, in dosages of 5 mg. (usually), and 10 mg. (occasionally), three or four times daily. Side effects were mild and transitory. Occurring singly, or in combination, they consisted of the following:

	Females	Males
Dizziness	2	1
Drowsiness: somnolence	8	4
Gastric distress: flatulence	1	--
Hypotension—slight	2	--
Lethargy	6	2
Muscular spasm—involving muscles of right shoulder	1	--
Xerostomia	7	1

During the study-period, prochlorperazine was the only internal agent prescribed for the relief of anxiety and tension (with consequent control of pruritus). Topical and actinic therapy were administered, as the condition of the patient warranted. All patients (drawn from private practice) were observed at weekly intervals, and study was pursued, without interruption, for intervals varying from four to 12 weeks. In eight patients, therapy was re-instituted as required, for the relief of tension, during intervals varying from 10-18 months. Urinalyses and hemograms were done on 14 patients, at monthly intervals, and all were within normal limits.

Drowsiness, somnolence and lethargy occurred in 20 patients, during the first week of therapy, clearing spontaneously in 12 patients as therapy continued. In eight patients, these side effects were disturbing enough to warrant concomitant administration of dextro-amphetamine sulfate.

In one female patient, who exhibited constriction of the shoulder muscles accompanied by acute pain (on a dosage of 10 mg. three times daily), there was clearance of this manifestation of reaction within a week after withdrawal of the drug.

In this series, we found neither objective nor subjective improvement in anxiety, nervousness and tension remarkable, and on the basis of our observations, our conclusion is that prochlorperazine has very limited application in dermatological therapy. Our impressions appear to confirm those of the Robinsons,[278] who reported observations of response (manifested by control of emotional tension) in 637 dermatological patients, following administration of various ataractic drugs. These investigators stated:

"Compazine. Each of 20 patients who were treated with Compazine had previously received hydroxyzine or meprobamate. Only 10 felt that this drug compared favorably with other medications."

Toxic Effects and Side Reactions

Dermal Reactions

Dermatitis 268

Allergic Phenomena

"Allergy-like manifestations" 268

Cardiovascular Complications

Hypotension 142, 268

Central Nervous System Effects

Dizziness: drowsiness: somnolence 142, 271
Excitomotor syndrome 68
Extrapyramidal involvement:
    Parkinsonism..68, 142, 260, 268, 270, 271
        In France, investigators[68] have reported peculiar manifestations, particularly associated with prochlorperazine.

These symptoms were acute and transitory and occurred without delay after administration of small doses of the drug. They were either of the excitomotor type, such as tremor, similar to that from a chill, myoclonia, sudden shaking with extension of the trunk, akathisia and tasikinesia, or of akinetic and occasionally of akinetohypertonic type with a fairly specific linguomasticatory and cervical localization. They were associated with a condition of psychomotor hypersuggestibility, causing them to be considered as "hysteroid." Oculogyric crises, similar to those which occur in patients with epidemic encephalitis were noted.

In Lesse's[142] series of 80 psychiatric patients (optimal dosage range 50 mg. to 60 mg. daily) four patients experienced extrapyramidal-like symptoms. One patient: stiffness of the face; another patient, when the daily dosage rose above 60 mg., said his tongue "felt clumsy."

Nasal congestion and xerostomia _____142, 271
Seizures _____266
Inasmuch as prochlorperazine is a phenothiazine derivative, "it should be administered discriminately, and patients should be observed carefully for toxic manifestations"_____260

PERPHENAZINE
(Trilafon—Schering Corporation)

Perphenazine is 1-(2-hydroxyethyl)-4-[3-(2-chloro-10-phenothiazyl)-propyl]-piperazine. The structural formula is shown, following:

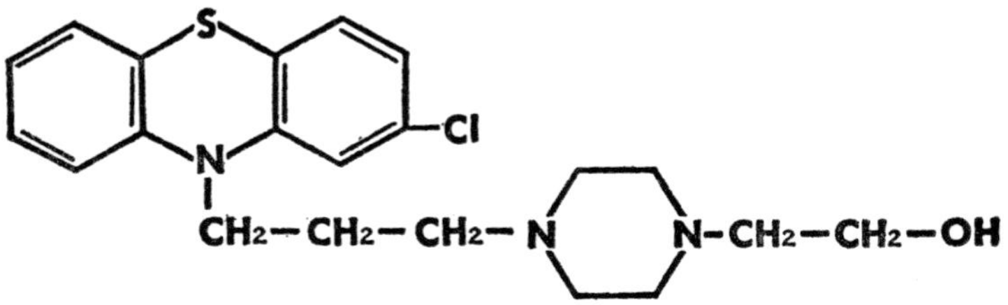

Pharmacologic Actions

The therapeutic index of perphenazine has been increased tenfold over that of chlorpromazine. Extensive pharmacologic studies in dogs, rats and mice have revealed that the LD_{50} of Trilafon is considerably higher than that of chlorpromazine; that is, by the several routes of administration in most species, perphenazine has proved to be approximately two-thirds as toxic as chlorpromazine. The oral lethal dose of the drug exceeded 100 mg./kg. in dogs. Hematologic studies, including blood sugar levels, hemoglobin hematocrit and nonprotein nitrogen were carried out in dogs, during a period of over six months. No abnormalities were found in any of the animals receiving the drug. Kidney and liver function tests in dogs, over a period of more than six months, showed consistently normal values. Routine urinalyses revealed no abnormalities. There was no significant tissue pathology following injections.

Perphenazine appears to possess five to ten times the behavioral potency of chlorpromazine, in various species, when administered by the several routes studied. Perphenazine also showed greater specificity of action on behavior than chlorpromazine.

Administration and Dosage

The dosage of perphenazine must be adjusted for each patient according to the severity of the condition and the response obtained. As with all potent drugs, the best dose is the lowest dose that will produce the desired clinical effect. It is very important to employ the lowest effective dose inasmuch as extrapyramidal symptoms increase in frequency and severity with increased dosage. Although these symptoms have disappeared upon reduction of dosage, withdrawal of the drug, or administration of benztropine methanesulfonate, it is believed at this time that prolonged administration of doses exceeding 24 mg. daily should be reserved for hospitalized patients. For simple anxiety and tension states, patients can be started on 2 mg. or 4 mg. three times daily. A total daily dosage of more than 16 mg. is seldom required to elicit a favorable response. For moderately disturbed outpatients, 4 mg. to 8 mg. three times daily during early management is suggested. Prompt reduction of dosage to minimum effective levels should be sought. The use of any dosage greater than 24 mg. daily should be avoided in ambulatory outpatients. Dosages for psychotic patients are higher, and are omitted from this discussion. Inasmuch as parenteral therapy is usually reserved for the treatment of acutely disturbed psychotics, dosage schedules are also omitted. They can be found in the manufacturer's literature.

General Clinical Uses

Perphenazine is indicated for the management of anxiety, tension and psychomotor hyperactivity in a wide variety of agitated mental and emotional disturbances, whether of functional origin, or associated with organic disorders.[14,124] The drug has been recommended for the management of anxiety, associated with organic disorders such as colitis, tension headache, intractable pruritus, dermatoses,[220] senility,[13,14] and arthritis; surgery;[168] protracted hiccups, drug withdrawal in addicts and intractable pain. The drug has also been recommended as an antiemetic for simple nausea and vomiting of pregnancy, and hyperemesis gravidarum; nausea and vomiting due to tension headaches; gastroenteritis, postoperative states, carcinomatosis, radiation therapy, psychogenic factors, or drugs.

The following statements are quoted from comments of Kinross-Wright[270] regarding piperazine phenothiazines:

"These have in common, a high potency—therapeutic doses averaging one-tenth of that of chlorpromazine, a slower onset of action, progressively increasing sedation (the reverse tends to be true for chlorpromazine) and a powerful action on the extrapyramidal system. Prochlorperazine (Compazine), trifluoroperazine (SKF 5019),* and perphenazine (Trilafon) are in this class. While essentially similar, the latter two drugs appear to be more successful therapeutically than Compazine."

Specific Dermatological Uses

Shanon[220] reported on response of 308 patients with various dermatoses complicated by psychogenic factors, treated with perphenazine for a period of five to seven weeks. Ages of the patients ranged from less than one year to 85 years. Dosages used were: 1 mg., 3 mg., 4 mg. and 8 mg. once, twice, thrice and four times daily.

A variety of dermatoses were included in his series, the major-

---

*SKF 5019, Smith Kline & French Laboratories, has not at this writing been marketed.

ity of cases being atopic dermatitis, neurodermatitis, urticaria, infantile eczema, eczematous hand dermatitis, seborrheic dermatitis, post-herpetic neuralgia, and pruritus ani et vulvae. There was no effect on pruritus, and there were no side effects, when patients were given 1 mg. to 3 mg. once or twice daily. In 144 patients with pruritis, who were given 4 mg. to 8 mg. two, three or four times daily, pruritus disappeared completely in 49 patients, and improved in 41 patients. In the psoriatic group, 41 out of 53 patients, when given perphenazine internally, and topical therapy with petrolatum, showed striking psychological "and initial skin improvement." Good results were also observed in atopic dermatitis and neurodermatitis, whereas in pruritis ani et vulvae, post-herpetic neuralgia and hand dermatitis, there was "no definite constant effect on itching."

Patch tests on 18 patients before, and after several weeks of therapy were negative after 48 to 72 hours, and no epidermal sensitization was observed.

Side effects usually appeared within 24 hours after taking the medication, the longest period between start of therapy and onset being two weeks.

The commonest side effects were:

> vertigo
> blurred vision
> drowsiness
> nausea
> dizziness
> excessive sweating
> shaking
> tension

Incidence of side effects was approximately 2%.

Certain extrapyramidal reactions were observed in four young patients who, when given 8 mg. four times daily, manifested symptoms "resembling conversion reactions." In all cases, symptoms disappeared promptly after therapy was discontinued or diminished. Symptoms consisted of stiffness of the neck and face, and thickness of the tongue.

Ten patients were hospitalized and intensively studied for a period of eight weeks, during perphenazine therapy. None devel-

oped agranulocytosis, jaundice, skin eruptions, bradycardia, tachycardia; there were no changes in blood pressure or in EEG and
EKG studies. These same patients were put into the sun, and no
photosensitivity cutaneous reactions developed.

Shanon's conclusion: "In general, the average dosage for dermatological patients should not exceed 8 mg. daily in adults, and
4 mg. in children and old people."

*

Kinross-Wright[270] cited the case of a male, aged 13 years,
treated for neurodermatitis. On a dosage of 4 mg. perphenazine
twice daily for three days, dystonia developed. (See pages 45-46 for
other comments.)

*

Study of perphenazine, as a tranquilizing agent in dermatological patients, was undertaken by the author and his associate in
September of 1956, and was pursued, without interruption, for an
interval of 20 months. All patients (a total of 558) were drawn from
private practice; all were observed at weekly intervals; and only
those who faithfully followed prescribed therapeutic regimens were
included in study-results. Perphenazine was the sole internal therapeutic agent administered for tranquilizing effect during the study
period; topical therapeutic regimens were varied as conditions
required; and actinic therapy was administered, as indicated. The
history of each patient was subjected to critical evaluation before
institution of perphenazine therapy, and patients having any symptoms, or history of liver dysfunction, or predisposition to seizures
were eliminated from inclusion in the study-group. Pertinent data,
such as normal hemograms, urinalyses, blood pressures and pulse
rates were recorded for comparative purposes.

The following table shows number of patients, age groups,
dosage schedules and diagnoses (in all of which there was some
strong psychogenic factor, either as a cause of the dermatological
disorder, or as a result of it).

After four consecutive weeks of therapy with perphenazine,
urinalyses and hemograms were obtained for 38 patients: monthly
urinalyses and hemograms were obtained for 24 patients, who

Diagnoses	Perphenazine 2 mg. two, three, four times daily		Perphenazine 4 mg. once, twice daily		Perphenazine 8 mg. once, twice daily	
	Females Ages 17-62	Males Ages 16-68	Females Ages 16-64	Males Ages 18-70	Females Ages 17-48	Males Ages 22-51
Acne: indurata	5	4	9	5	4	2
rosacea	4	2	5	7	--	--
vulgaris	2	2	--	--	--	--
Alopecia	8	6	12	8	4	1
Angioneurotic edema: urticaria	5	--	10	8	--	--
Atopic dermatitis	18	8	24	18	6	4
Chronic infectious eczematoid dermatitis	22	16	22	16	4	2
Contact dermatitis	14	9	17	11	6	4
Dermatitis herpetiformis	1	1	--	--	--	--
Dermatitis medicamentosa	4	2	4	2	--	--
Hyperhidrosis	7	4	5	4	--	--
Lichen planus	4	--	12	1	--	--
Lichen sclerosus et atrophicus	4	--	8	2	--	--
Lupus erythematosus: subacute disseminated	--	--	2	--	--	--
chronic discoid	1	--	1	--	--	--
Neurodermatitis	8	1	12	2	6	--
Pruritus ani et vulvae	5	7	10	6	4	2
Psoriasis	6	4	12	10	6	4
Seborrheic dermatitis	8	7	18	10	--	--
Stasis dermatitis	4	1	2	1	--	--
Totals	129	74	185	111	40	19
Grand Total					558	

received the drug for seven months. All studies were within normal limits.

The longest interval of treatment was seven months: the shortest, three days: the average duration of therapy, three months.

Toxic manifestations and side reactions to therapy, observed singly or in combination, in descending order of frequency, were the following, occurring in 99 patients in our series:

	Number of Manifestations of Reaction
Drowsiness: somnolence: lethargy	27
Gastric distress	23

Generalized weakness 19
Xerostomia, severe enough to evoke complaint .. 16
Disturbance of menstrual cycle 10
Paradoxical excitement and irritability 8
Dysphagia 3
Dermatitis 2
Syncope 2
Photophobia 1

All manifestations of reaction observed by us were reversible, when medication was withdrawn: none was serious, the extrapyramidal manifestations causing us (and the patients) most concern. In one patient (a female, aged 34 years) paradoxical excitement and irritability persisted for five days after withdrawal of medication. One female patient, aged 30 years, experienced boardlike rigidity of the tongue, difficulty in talking, dysphagia, and severe "burning of the eyes," with onset of symptoms on the third day of medication: dosage 12 mg. daily. Medication was withdrawn. Difficult speech continued until the ninth day thereafter. Eye symptoms subsided completely on the sixth day, and diagnosis of ocular symptoms by an ophthalmologist was photophobia. Other phenothiazine derivatives have occasionally been known to induce photophobia.[185, 239] Another female patient, aged 19 years, experienced rigidity of the tongue and dysphagia on the tenth day of therapy, on a dosage of perphenazine, 8 mg. daily. Medication was withdrawn and two days later, symptoms subsided.

A maculopapular eruption over the forearms appeared in one female patient on the eighth day of therapy: daily dosage, 4 mg. The eruption cleared in three days, following withdrawal of medication.

One female patient, aged 71 years, on a dosage of 4 mg. daily, returned for observation one week following institution of therapy. She said she had taken her medication for four days, and "palpitations" alarmed her, so she stopped. When observed, her blood pressure and pulse rate were normal. We did not think it wise to urge another trial of the drug, and we have not included this case in our series of manifestations of reaction.

We attribute the two cases of syncope to hypotensive episodes, inasmuch as we have observed such episodes produced by other tranquilizing agents.[250]

Forty of the 99 patients experiencing reactions were arbitrarily maintained for six weeks on placebo therapy, after one month of perphenazine therapy—the patients having no knowledge of change in medication. Thirty-eight of those patients (with side effects while on the active preparation) experienced disappearance of side effects while on the placebo.

Response of patients with hyperhidrosis was uniformly good to treatment with Trilapran (a combination of perphenazine 4 mg. and diphemanil methylsulfate, Prantal Methylsulfate, 200 mg.), administered once or twice daily (rarely, three times daily). Some of our younger patients, afflicted with excessive sweating, found that by taking Trilapran just before "going out," or making a public appearance, embarrassment might be avoided. From our observations, we conclude that such combination of therapeutic agents is more effective, for the control of excessive sweating, than either agent, alone.

Control of pruritus by perphenazine appeared to be determined by individual response to medication. We found that such control seemed to fluctuate, both qualitatively and quantitatively, in the same individual. We consider that about 70% of our patients experienced reduction of tension and general calming effect, during perphenazine therapy. Their dermatoses were not so much improved—patients simply bore them more tolerantly, and more comfortably.

We observed that six patients with seborrheic dermatitis manifested decided flares of their lesions during perphenazine therapy. Such exacerbations may have been seasonal, or coincidental, but we, and other investigators,[165] have observed similar response to other phenothiazine derivatives.

We consider perphenazine to have a certain usefulness for the management of anxiety, tension and pruritus (which are exacerbating factors in various dermatoses). We think it important, however, that dermatologists be aware of the "potential for harm" inherent to varying degrees in all phenothiazine derivatives, of which perphenazine is one.

Toxic Effects and Side Reactions

Dermal Reactions

Marangoni described a series of 60 (hospitalized) patients with anxiety and tension treated with Trilafon,
wherein the minimum effective levels of dosage were between 12 mg. and 14 mg. daily. Side effects developed in
two patients: in one, an allergic skin reaction, which
cleared when the dosage was reduced. This patient had
had an allergic response several months earlier, during

(See page 43)

Cardiovascular Complications

(See pages 43-44)

Central Nervous System Effects

According to Kinross-Wright . . . "incidence with Trilafon is 50%. This is also true of Compazine and SKF
5019. With these drugs, Parkinsonism appears with doses
of 30 mg. daily and up, varying of course greatly in different individuals. It is always reversible upon reducing
dosage or discontinuing the drug. The disorder is characterized by rigidity, some tremor, salivation, masking of the
face, and gait difficulties. Onset is frequently preceded
by several days of restlessness and feelings of tension."

In addition to the above, Kinross-Wright pointed out
that Trilafon produces two other neuromuscular abnormalities:

1. Dystonic symptoms, or torsion spasm, which may
precede or develop independently of Parkinsonism.

2. Dysphagia, without Parkinsonism or dystonia. Upon
examination, there is found localized rigidity of the
tongue and pharyngeal muscles, without actual incoordi-
nation of the swallowing mechanism.

He cited the case of a 12-year-old girl, who developed
spasm of the left neck muscles and shoulder girdle after a

single dose of 4 mg. "It sometimes has an explosive onset and may be almost epileptic in appearance."

Other investigators have reported extrapyramidal dysfunction_____13, 220, 260, 271

(See page 43)

Dreams and nightmares _____13, 271
Drowsiness (persistent) _____220, 270
Dysphagia   (See page 43)
Miosis _____13, 271
Muscular aches and pains (neuromuscular
   abnormalities)_____13, 14, 271
Photophobia   (See page 43)
Vertigo: dizziness _____220
Vision-blurring _____220
Sweating _____220
Tension: paradoxical excitement _____220

(See page 43)

Endocrine Imbalances

Experiments have revealed that Trilafon is effective in inducing pseudo-pregnancy in adult rats of known regular estrous history. After drug withdrawal, the animals returned to their normal estrous cycles _____242
In the Kinross-Wright report on treatment of 37 psychotic patients, lactation developed in one patient. This investigator says: "We have noted it with several of the phenothiazines" _____270
Disturbance of menstrual cycle_____ (See page 43)

Gastrointestinal Disturbances

Constipation _____13
Gastric distress: nausea _____220, 270

(See page 42)

TRIMEPRAZINE
(*Temaril*—Smith Kline & French Laboratories)

Trimeprazine is dl-10-(3-dimethylamino-2-methylpropyl) phenothiazine. Structural formula for the tartrate salt is shown, following:

$$CH_2-CH-CH_2N(CH_3)_2$$
$$CH_3$$

$$\cdot COOH-CHOH-CHOH-COOH$$
$$2$$

Pharmacologic Actions

According to the Investigational Use Circular, supplied by the manufacturers, acute toxicity studies in mice revealed LD_{50} values, following oral and intravenous administration, which were comparable to those of chlorpromazine. In protecting against histamine-induced bronchospasm in the guinea-pig, trimeprazine was found to be considerably more active than promethazine (Phenergan). Trimeprazine was found to be about one-third as potent as chlorpromazine in blocking the response to a conditioned reflex in rats. Reduction of spontaneous motor activity in mice is used as a measure of the central depressant activity of a drug. In this test, trimeprazine had about one-half the activity of chlorpromazine.

Administration and Dosage

For adults, the usual dosage is 2.5 mg. twice daily after meals, plus 5 mg., at bedtime. Generally, 10 mg. during 24 hours represents optimal dosage. In cases where itching is primarily a nighttime problem, doses of 5 mg. to 10 mg. at bedtime may be effective without supplementary daytime doses. When the nighttime dose carries the patient through the following morning, daytime doses should be administered after lunch and after supper. Otherwise, daytime doses should be administered after breakfast and after lunch. Some patients may require 20 mg. to 30 mg. during 24 hours, and in non-ambulatory patients with severe pruritus, as much as 80 mg. during 24 hours has been used. For children, relief may be obtained with 2.5 mg. at bedtime. If daytime therapy is required, one or two 2.5 mg. doses may be administered, after meals.

General Clinical Uses

Trimeprazine is recommended for the treatment of pruritus, regardless of etiology. Preliminary clinical impressions, rather than final conclusions, suggest efficacy of the drug for dermatoses wherein relief of pruritus is the therapeutic objective; for the treatment of respiratory allergies; for symptomatic relief of conditions associated with muscle spasm; for the treatment of psychoses and psychoneuroses.

Specific Dermatological Uses

According to the Investigational Use Circular supplied by the manufacturers, early clinical studies indicated the following:

Dose response in dermatological patients:
86% in patients on 5 mg. to 30 mg. daily
82% in patients on 40 mg. to 90 mg. daily
50% in patients on 100 mg. to 200 mg. daily

Drowsiness was the most frequently-encountered side effect, occurring in 60% of all patients, excluding those with psychoses. With reduced dosage (retaining therapeutic effectiveness), this manifestation of reaction decreased or disappeared. Other patients "developed tolerance to drowsiness, in one or two weeks, when the drug was continued at the same, or higher doses." The administration of amphetamine, concomitantly, allowed some patients to continue with daytime medication. One case of dermatitis was definitely attributable to the drug—and one other case "may" have been caused by it.

In the more than 1,200 patients treated with the drug, one case of agranulocytosis had been reported.

Side effects observed in 285 patients were:

Symptom or Sign	Number of	Times Seen
Somnolence (all degrees)	171	60%
Somnolence (severe)	34	12
Dryness of the mucous membranes	34	12
Dizziness	27	9
Nausea and/or vomiting	7	2.5
Nightmares	6	2.1

Generalized weakness	5	1.7
Fainting	3	1.0
Dermatitis	2	0.3

Experience of the University of Pennsylvania group[180] with trimeprazine was as follows: the drug was administered to some 300 patients, from whom follow-up reports on administration for periods as long as 10 months made possible analysis of response by 200 patients. The conditions treated included all types of pruritic dermatitic and eczematous eruptions, with atopic dermatitis, localized neurodermatitis, and severe anal and vulvar pruritis in the majority; and a few cases of infantile and childhood eczema; lichen planus, urticaria, contact dermatitis, dermatitis herpetiformis and senile pruritis.

These observers found trimeprazine to be the only systemically-administered compound, aside from the corticosteroids and antihistamines, in certain selected cases, which has a definite, reasonably regular antipuritic effect. The exact degree of efficacy, however, was difficult to evaluate. It was estimated that in 70% of this series, relief of itching was good-to-excellent, that is, of a degree sufficient to make the compound worthwhile. In those patients, who showed no response, it was possible that an increase in dose would have yielded some result. Such increase was impossible in outpatients, because of the fairly regular sedative effects of larger doses.

In hospitalized patients, doses of 10 mg. to 25 mg. four times daily could be given (during which the patients slept almost continuously). Experiments with outpatients led to diminution of initial dose to determine at which level sedative effects were not bothersome. These investigators considered the question as to whether sedative effects were related to antipruritic effects, and concluded that the two have no direct relationship; inasmuch as many patients have excellent relief from pruritus without apparent sedation.

No untoward effects to therapy were noted, either cutaneous or hepatic. Hematologic study in 50 patients, who had taken the compound continuously for two or more weeks, demonstrated no significant changes. An occasional patient complained of mild gastrointestinal upset, or dryness of the mouth, but these reactions did not necessitate withdrawal of medication. One patient developed mild photosensitivity on the forehead, after prolonged exposure at the seashore, although he was subsequently able to tolerate exposure to strong sunlight.

The final statement of the report: " . . the tranquilizing action of trimeprazine cannot be expected to occur regularly, as it does with rauwolfia, meprobamate or chlorpromazine."

*

Callaway and Olansky[45] treated 85 patients suffering from various dermatoses, in which pruritus was the most prominent symptom. Trimeprazine was used in an average dosage of 10 mg. daily. Response was considered "excellent" if complete relief from itching resulted: "good," if itching was considerably reduced: "fair," if some reduction of itching was obtained: and "poor," if pruritus was unaffected. Seventy patients (82%) obtained excellent-to-good results. In 39 patients with atopic eczema, excellent results were obtained in eight; good, in 23; and fair, in eight. There were no failures. Seven children, aged six to 15 years, whose pruritus was caused by chickenpox, obtained marked relief from an average dose of 5 mg. twice or three times daily. Children were given the drug as syrup, 1 mg. per ml. (0.5 teaspoonful) four times daily. The only side effect noted in this series was drowsiness, which, in many patients, subsided as medication was continued; or was overcome by adjustment of dosage.

*

Study of trimeprazine was undertaken, August 1, 1957, by the author and his associate in order to further broaden experience and widen knowledge regarding phenothiazine psychotherapeutic drugs. All patients were selected from private practice: all were observed at weekly intervals. Trimeprazine was the sole internal therapeutic agent administered for antipruritic and sedative effect during the study period: topical therapeutic regimens being varied as conditions required, and actinic therapy being administered, where indicated. The same patient-screening procedure was followed for this study, as for the study on perphenazine (see page 41).

The following table shows number of patients, age groups,

dosage schedules and diagnoses (in all of which there was some strong psychogenic factor, either as a cause of the dermatological disorder, or as a result of it).

Diagnosis	Trimeprazine 2.5 mg. two, three, four times daily		Trimeprazine 5 mg. two, three, four times daily		Trimeprazine 10 mg. two, three times daily	
	Females Ages 12-66	Males Ages 15-58	Females Ages 17-61	Males Ages 19-58	Females Ages 22-61	Males Ages 31-70
Angioneurotic edema: urticaria	5	--	4	2	--	--
Atopic dermatitis	28	5	9	3	--	--
Chronic infectious eczematoid dermatitis	20	8	11	4	6	4
Contact dermatitis	22	7	14	6	3	2
Dermatitis herpetiformis	2	--	--	1	—	—
Dermatitis medicamentosa	1	1	2	--	—	--
Epidermophytosis	--	3	--	2	—	1
Intertrigo	4	2	7	3	--	--
Lichen planus	8	2	6	1	—	—
Miliaria	6	3	4	1	--	--
Neurodermatitis	21	9	16	2	10	--
Pruritus ani et vulvae	19	7	16	5	8	2
Psoriasis	8	4	7	3	--	--
Schamberg's disease	--	--	--	1	--	--
Seborrheic dermatitis	7	5	6	4	--	--
Stasis dermatitis	13	3	11	4	7	4
Totals	164	59	113	42	34	13
Grand Total						425

After two weeks of consecutive therapy, urinalyses and hemograms were obtained on 24 patients: after four weeks, on 41 patients: monthly urinalyses and hemograms were obtained on 46 patients undergoing therapy for intervals of nine and 10 months. No abnormalities were noted.

The longest interval of treatment was 10 months: the shortest, 10 days: the average, 6 months, consecutively; 10 months, intermittently.

Our evaluation of response to medication was based on increase or decrease in excoriations and/or erythema; and on subjective improvement or lack of it, reported by the patient. These are the manifestations (of failure of trimeprazine to control pruritis, and reaction to therapy), appearing either singly, or in combination, in descending order of frequency, in 261 patients, during our study.

	Number of Manifestations
Increased excoriations, indicative of uninhibited scratching	96
Drowsiness: somnolence	88
Dizziness	26
Gastric distress	18
Generalized weakness	15
Xerostomia, severe enough to evoke complaints	8
Dermatitis	1
Syncope	1

The following is quoted from the Investigational Use Circular supplied by Smith Kline & French Laboratories,

" . . . patients developed tolerance to drowsiness . . . "

In our opinion, tolerance to drowsiness means that the patient is developing tolerance to the medication, which no longer makes him drowsy. In 20 of our patients, who did not develop sufficient "tolerance to drowsiness," after two weeks of therapy, concomitant administration of dextro-amphetamine sulfate was required.

All manifestations of reaction were reversible, when medication was withdrawn: none was serious. Fifty-five individuals (chosen from the group of 261 patients manifesting either failure of trimeprazine to control pruritus, or reaction to therapy) were arbitrarily maintained for a month on placebo therapy, after at least one month of trimeprazine therapy (the patients having no knowledge of change in medication). Forty-eight of those subjects (with side effects other than uncontrolled pruritus) experienced disappearance of side effects while on the placebo.

Results of our study indicate that trimeprazine is most useful in patients having atopic dermatitis, neurodermatitis, contact dermatitis and lichen planus. The drug seemed to enable those patients to resume and maintain normal sleep-habits. In our series of patients, pruritis was controlled effectively in approximately 55%, and was not controlled in approximately 45% of cases. When trimeprazine was discontinued (in those patients having control of pruritus, or reduction of it) symptoms promptly recurred in 48% of cases. Recurrence of symptoms, following discontinuation of therapy with other phenothiazine derivatives has been reported by other investigators.[60] Symptoms could be relieved by resumption of medication.

In our experience, it would appear that, in certain patients, tolerance develops to the antipruritic effects as well as to the sedative effects of trimeprazine. (After repeated administration, tolerance has been reported to develop to chlorpromazine, particularly to the hypotensive and hypnotic effects.[166]) We found that this characteristic of trimeprazine required, for many patients having problems of long duration, either that the drug be stopped for a few days (which cannot well be done when pruritus is prolonged and severe), or that the dosage be increased.

We observed no hematopoietic changes; no cardiovascular complications: no allergic phenomena, such as photosensitivity, or toxic liver changes. We were, however, disappointed with response of our patients to trimeprazine therapy. That our disappointment is shared, is well expressed in the following:[245,246]

"I continue to be somewhat disappointed in the effectiveness of this drug as regards to itching. I do think it is an excellent tranquilizer, however, even in those cases where it does not relieve the itching. In summary, I should say then that I think this drug has been somewhat overrated in the initial reports; however, I still feel that there are certain areas of treatment where it is useful."

To summarize: we consider that trimeprazine has some use for the control of pruritus, in certain patients, particularly those with acute atopic dermatitis, neurodermatitis, contact dermatitis, chronic infectious eczematoid dermatitis and lichen planus. We point out, however, that certain other antipruritic agents, such as the antihistamines (particularly antihistamines with mild, sedative effects) do not possess the "potential for harm" which is an inherent characteristic of the phenothiazine derivatives. We think it important for dermatologists to weigh possible benefits against this potential before prescribing any psychotherapeutic agents of the phenothiazine group.

Toxic Effects and Side Reactions

Dermal Reactions

Dermatitis_____(See pages 49, 52)

    The author has been advised, by Dr. Lawrence G. Beinhauer, of a case of giant urticaria, which developed in a female patient within 24 hours after ingestion of 10 mg. of trimeprazine (the only internal medication administered for the control of pruritus, associated with neurodermatitis involving the back of the neck, eyelids and vulva). Lesions resolved on the fourth day, following withdrawal of the drug. It was deemed inadvisable to administer trimeprazine to the patient, a second time.

Photosensitivity (?)_____(See page 50)

Cardiovascular Complications

Fainting and generalized weakness, as possible
    manifestation of hypotension_____(See pages 49 and 52)

Central Nervous System Effects

Dizziness _____(See pages 48 and 52)
Dreams: nightmares_____(See page 48)
Drowsiness: somnolence_____(See pages 48-50, 52)

Gastrointestinal Disturbances

Gastric distress_____(See pages 48-49, 52)

Hematopoietic Changes

Agranulocytosis _____(See page 48)

Section II

Rauwolfia – Alkaloids and Fractions

RAUWOLFIA — ALKALOIDS AND FRACTIONS

Powdered Whole Root of
Rauwolfia serpentina (Benth.)   Raudixin

Alseroxylon   Rauwiloid

Reserpine   Serpasil

Rescinnamine   Moderil

Recanescine   Harmonyl

RAUWOLFIA — ALKALOIDS AND FRACTIONS

Among the tropical trees and shrubs of the dogbane family are the rauwolfia species (named after the German doctor, botanist and traveler, Leonhard Rauwolf[194]). There are two important species (medicinally speaking): Rauwolfia serpentina Benth. and Rauwolfia canescens Linn. (although there are more than 131 species of Rauwolfia distributed in tropical regions throughout the world, and eight varieties are reported to occur in India). Since antiquity, preparations of the root of Rauwolfia serpentina (Benth.) have been used by native practioners as an antidote to snakebite, as a vermifuge, as an antipyretic, and to allay the psychomotor hyperactivity in neuropsychiatric disorders.[183] It was in 1933 that Indian scientists observed and reported the antihypertensive action of rauwolfia (the name now given to the powdered whole root of the plant).

RAUWOLFIA—POWDERED WHOLE ROOT OF RAUWOLFIA SERPENTINA (BENTH.) N.N.D.

(Example: *Raudixin*—E. R. Squibb & Sons)

Pharmacologic Actions

The powdered whole root of Rauwolfia serpentina (Benth.) produces the sum of the actions of the total alkaloids contained in the whole root. The component alkaloids exhibit the sedative-antihypertensive-bradycrotic action characteristic of reserpine, the latter of which accounts for 50% of their total activity. The whole root contains only insignificant amounts of yohimbine and other adrenolytic alkaloids. Thus rauwolfia is useful for the same purposes, and with the same precautions as for reserpine.[166]

Administration and Dosage

Rauwolfia is administered orally. For adults, the average dosage: 200 mg. to 400 mg. daily, in divided doses. Larger doses may be required for sedation of gross psychotic disturbances than for anxiety-tension states, associated with mild, labile hypertension. (Orally, 200 mg. to 300 mg. of powdered whole root is equivalent to 0.5 mg. reserpine.[166])

ALSEROXYLON N.N.D.
(Example: *Rauwiloid*—Riker Laboratories)

Alseroxylon is a fat-soluble alkaloidal fraction extracted from the root of Rauwolfia serpentina (Benth.), containing reserpine and other non-adrenolytic amorphous alkaloids.[166]

Pharmacologic Actions

Alseroxylon has the action of the sedative-antihypertensive-bradycrotic alkaloids of Rauwolfia serpentina, of which reserpine is among the most potent. It has the same uses and limitations as the whole root, rauwolfia, and its chief component alkaloid, reserpine.

Administration and Dosage

Alseroxylon is administered orally. For adults, the average dose: 2 mg. to 4 mg. daily. Higher oral dosage may be required for sedation of gross psychotic disturbances than for anxiety-tension syndromes associated with mild, labile hypertension. (Orally, 1 mg. is approximately equivalent to 0.2 mg. of reserpine.[166])

RESERPINE N.N.D.
(Example: *Serpasil*—Ciba Pharmaceutical Products, Inc.)

Reserpine is an ester alkaloid, isolated in 1952 in Switzerland, from the root of certain species of rauwolfia. The structural formula is shown, following:

Pharmacologic Actions

Reserpine is considered to be one of the most potent of the rauwolfia alkaloids, which exhibit a sedative action and antihypertensive effect, accompanied by bradycardia. Its antihypertensive effect is variable and ineffective in some patients. Studies in experimental animals indicate that the drug acts upon the central nervous system, producing a psychotherapeutic nonhypnotic sedation, ptosis of the eyelids, sinus bradycardia, increased secretory and motor activity of the gastrointestinal tract, and a variable lowering of mean arterial blood pressure. The latter effect is attributed to a decrease in peripheral vasoconstriction, apparently induced by central action on the vasomotor mechanism, and is not associated with a significant alteration of cardiac output or renal plasma flow.[166] Some effects of the drug suggest an action on the autonomic nervous system, although it does not exhibit either peripheral adrenolytic or peripheral parasympathomimetic activity, and it does not block autonomic ganglions. Its observed effects are presumed to result from a central partial suppression of sympathetic predominance near the level of the hypothalamus, where autonomic nervous functions are integrated.[119]

Recent evidence suggests that tranquilizing action may be mediated through serotonin, which is a naturally-occurring constituent of nervous tissue. According to Pletscher *et al.*,[182] the serotonin concentration in the brain stem of rabbits is about three times that of the remainder of the brain; studies on animals suggesting that rauwolfia alkaloids exert effect by modifying serotonin activity. A short time after administration, reserpine can no longer be found in the brain, although serotonin-binding inhibition may persist for as long as 48 hours. These observations support the postulation that serotonin may function as a neurohumoral synaptic transmitter, and may act, primarily, in the hypothalamic area as a mediator of inhibitory nerve impulses. At this writing only three of the alkaloids of rauwolfia (reserpine, rescinnamine and recanescine) are considered to have action on serotonin, and they are the only alkaloids having tranquilizing effect.

Administration and Dosage

Reserpine may be administered orally, and parenterally. For anxiety-tension and related disorders, the initial daily dose range is 0.1 mg. to 0.5 mg. Since individualization of dosage is necessary for optimal results, initial dose should be adjusted according to the patient's response. As little as 0.1 mg. daily is often sufficient for maintenance. It may be given as a single dose, or in divided doses. Dosage schedules for psychiatric conditions, alcoholism, hypertension, tachycardia and the like are omitted from this discussion. They may be obtained from the manufacturer's literature.

Variations of action appear to be more a function of dosage and individual responsiveness, than of route of administration. With daily oral administration, effects of the drug, usually, are not fully manifest for several days to two weeks, and may persist for as long as four weeks after oral medication is discontinued. Tolerance to the drug does not develop with continued administration.[166]

General Clinical Uses

Reserpine is useful, chiefly, for its psychotherapeutic sedative action in the symptomatic management of patients with anxiety or tension, psychoneuroses as such, or as an accompaniment to somatic disorders, and of patients with chronic psychoses involving anxiety, psychomotor hyperactivity or compulsive aggressive behavior.[166] It is useful, also, for management of mild, labile hypertension associated with anxiety and emotional factors, and in conjunction with potent hypotensive agents for the management of essential hypertension and hypertension associated with toxemia of pregnancy.[166] The use of the drug alone is considered to be of little value for severe or fixed hypertension, but it is useful to enhance or prolong the action of potent hypotensive agents, to reduce dosage, and side effects. It probably should not be used with barbiturates, particularly in conditions in which profound sedation would be undesirable.[166]

In patients with grossly-disturbed psychoses, and in patients with anxiety-tension states, the drug must be administered for a period of one (usually), or two weeks, before the optimal level of dosage can be determined.[166]

Specific Dermatological Uses

Rein and Goodman[192] undertook one of the early studies for evaluation of the tranquilizing and relaxing effects of reserpine in a selected group of 60 patients, with various dermatoses, in whom there was uncontrollable urge to scratch, or in whom a factor of nervous tension contributed to the cutaneous disorders. The dosage was 0.25 mg. four times daily for one month. Patients were re-examined at weekly intervals, and questioned as to subjective sensations. Blood pressure and pulse were recorded each time.

It was noted that patients experienced moderate drowsiness and fatigue starting, usually, from the second to fourth days after onset of therapy. These symptoms gradually subsided during the second week. Of the 60 patients, 40 experienced definite relaxation, tranquilization and sedation, and lessening of tension. There was no significant blood pressure or pulse change in this essentially normotensive group. Patients with palmar hyperhidrosis, within two weeks, experienced a decided reduction in the degree of hyperhidrosis.

Side reactions, none of which was considered serious, were:

	Number of Patients
Nasal congestion	24
Increased appetite	13
Dreams	8
Nocturia	8

Therapy was discontinued in five subjects during the first week because of marked fatigue, drowsiness and weakness: in two patients with asthmatic backgrounds, because of moderate dyspnea: in two patients who developed nausea, and in one patient because of moderate depression. (These patients were not included in the total of 60 patients evaluated.)

Thirty patients were arbitrarily maintained a month or so on placebo therapy, after one month of reserpine (the patients not being notified of the change). All patients with side effects, while on the active preparation noted that these side effects disappeared on the placebo. In general, it was noted that the effects of reserpine wore off by the end of two weeks, after the drug had been discontinued. In seven patients, however, there was reserpine-effect extending beyond the two weeks of placebo therapy.

Rein and Goodman reviewed the work of Lenahan and Kesten; stated that continued experience with a series of more than 300 dermatological patients proved to be similar to response observed in the original 60 patients; called attention to the work of Freis,[96] and stated the belief that the maintenance dose of reserpine in dermatological patients should be kept below 0.25 mg. daily (in order to minimize possible development of psychotic symptoms).

*

Ferrara and Pinkus[87] reported observation of response following use of alseroxylon (Rauwiloid) by 36 patients with pruritic and psychogenic dermatoses. These patients experienced definite, but varying degrees of relaxation, tranquilization and mild sedation. Pruritus was relieved or decreased to varying degrees in all patients, except one with urticaria. They found that in general, side effects were of little importance in all patients, except in one, who complained of marked fatigue; that these side effects included the following:

> fatigue and drowsiness
> nasal congestion
> increased appetite and weight gain
> dreams, thirst, nocturia

*

Other investigators[141, 260, 263, 265, 271, 274, 278] have reported on the control of emotional tension in dermatoses in patients treated with rauwolfia and various derivatives thereof.

Toxic Effects and Side Reactions

Dermal Reactions

Newman[167] reported petechial eruptions, and the appearance of essential purpura simplex, appearing in a number of patients, who had been on rauwolfia derivatives for prolonged intervals. He concluded:

> "Of course, there is nothing unusual in untoward reactions
> to drugs developing after long periods of use. However, the
> development of an insidious eruption, barely perceptible, grad-

ually spreading and increasing in intensity over many months is a unique experience."

Ross[199] reported a toxic eruption, in a patient with psoriasis, on reserpine therapy 0.25 mg. twice daily for one month (with improvement in her temperament, if not in her psoriasis), and on 0.25 mg. daily for a period of six and one-half months. A generalized petechial eruption brought the patient to his attention—the eruption developing into hemorrhagic and ecchymotic areas. Upon cessation of medication, the entire eruption disappeared. It was deemed unwise to have the patient repeat the drug.

There have been other reports of development of a hemorrhagic diathesis, with thrombopenia, in patients who had received therapy with reserpine.[205]

*

Panaccio[173] observed generalized eczematous dermatitis. Other investigators have mentioned allergic dermatitis, rash with pruritus, and urticaria.[93, 111, 227, 249, 259, 262]

*

There have been numerous reports of generalized skin flushing and conjunctival injection, attributable to the vasodilator effects of rauwolfia.[71, 105, 119, 120, 154, 259]

Troublesome nasal stuffiness and epistaxis have been observed:[1, 6, 30, 71, 80, 87, 119, 128, 153, 154, 193, 249, 259, 262, 265, 278] also hyperthermia:[259] undue susceptibility to cold.[1, 71, 259] These effects have been attributed to peripheral vasodilatation from central inhibition of the sympathetic nervous system; and possible direct action on the blood vessel wall.

Reserpine has a definite effect in the newborn infant of mothers, who received the drug prior to delivery (probably due to rapid accumulation of the drug in the infant via the placenta).[41, 197] The severity of toxic symptoms and nasal discharge appeared without any correlation between amount of drug administered to the mother, time of onset and severity of symptoms in the infant. Postmortem examination of a newborn infant revealed a generalized vascular dilatation of the capillaries and venules, which might be a secondary effect of anoxia, a result of the drug alone, or a result of both factors.

A fixed drug eruption has been reported,[65] in one case, follow-

ing therapy with Serpasil. The eruption appeared in the antecu-
bital fossae, symmetrically distributed, and at a later date, was reproduced by administration of the offending drug. The author and his
associate have observed two cases of fixed drug eruptions, which
occurred on the flexor surfaces of the forearms, and which could be
reproduced by repeated administration of reserpine.

Various other toxic effects and side reactions are summarized,
in the following:

Allergic Phenomena

Asthmatiform paroxysm with facial edema
   and congestion _____173, 177
Diaphoresis _____259
Edema _____259

Cardiovascular Complications

Bradycardia and tachycardia _____259
     Surgical hypertensive patients on rauwolfia therapy
    have shown significant hypotension and bradycardia dur-
    ing anesthesia _____53, 128
     Electrocardiographic tracings have shown ischemic
    myocardial changes. There are significant circulatory
    changes. Patients on rauwolfia therapy, who are to un-
    dergo elective surgery, should not receive the drug for two
    weeks prior to surgical procedures. Emergency surgery on
    these patients may be safely carried out by using vagal
    blocking agents, such as atropine sulfate, scopolamine or
    oxyphenonium, to prevent and treat vagal circulatory
    responses.
Edema and congestive heart failure _____177
Hypotension (orthostatic), appearing frequently, after paren-
    teral administration; more rarely, after oral administra-
    tion, except with large dosages. There may be numbness
    and tingling of the extremities: and syncope_____6, 93, 94, 259
Premature ventricular contractions_____207, 253
     Physicians should be alerted to the fact that rauwolfia
    therapy may produce premature ventricular contractions
    in all patients, but more readily, in digitalized patients.

Central Nervous System Effects

Agitated or paranoid depression, with
   suicidal tendencies........1, 71, 80, 94, 96, 146, 164, 208, 273, 278
Dizziness 6, 105, 128, 153, 259
Dreams..1, 6, 87, 93, 128, 249, 259
Drowsiness: sedation....1, 24, 30, 71, 80, 87, 120, 128, 146, 154, 265
Euphoria 93, 128
Fatigue and weakness........6, 71, 87, 93, 94, 120, 128, 153, 259, 265
Headache 1, 30
Insomnia: nervousness..93, 193
Miosis 154
Muscular aches and pains........................1, 30, 193, 259, 278
Paradoxical anxiety..93, 193
Parkinsonism........................6, 24, 40, 93, 120, 153, 193, 259, 273
Seizures: Grand-mal in type, in patients with no history
   of convulsive disorders..208, 273
Urinary frequency and urgency..1, 87, 249
   Thirst
Xerostomia 6, 93, 193, 259

Endocrine Imbalances

Erotic behavior..6
Inhibition of androgen secretion, by the testis, in humans........100
   According to one investigator: "The slowness of action
   of the drugs (rauwolfia) has suggested that they work
   through some hormonal or other intermediate mechanism. One hormonal route readily and currently suggested is the adrenal cortex, particularly through the sex-
   stimulating steroids. There is some clinical evidence for
   this in men, who uniformly comment, if not complain,
   about a decrease in libido while taking the drug. This,
   however, is definitely not impotence, and two young men
   have fathered new babies while on the drug"........................123
Modification of the menstrual cycle
   in animals..21, 22, 66, 67
   and in humans 100
Reduction of basal metabolic rate in euthyroidal experimen-
   tal subjects. It has been postulated that reserpine has
   beneficial effects upon the clinical manifestations of
   hyperthyroidism, possibly by altering the reaction of the

body to excessive thyroid hormone, or by counteracting
the effects of the hormone on body cells........................47
Sodium retention, and development of edema................177
   This mechanism of reaction is obscure. It has been
postulated that reserpine may stimulate release of the anti-
diuretic hormone.

Gastrointestinal Disturbances

Anorexia 1, 6, 30
Constipation 153
Diarrhea: increased number of bowel
   movements...1, 6, 71, 80, 87, 93, 105, 128, 146, 153, 154, 193, 259
"Discomfort" 105
Excessive appetite and weight gain................1, 80, 87, 93, 249
Gastrointestinal hyperactivity, including increased gastric
   secretion, reactivation of peptic ulcers, and gastric hemor-
   rhage 6, 193, 201, 221
Nausea and vomiting................6, 30, 146, 249, 259

RESCINNAMINE

(Moderil—Chas. Pfizer & Company, Inc.)

Rescinnamine is the 3, 4, 5-trimethoxycinnamic acid ester of
methyl reserpate. The compound is shown, by the following structural formula:

Pharmacologic Actions

In 1954, renewed attempts to extract and identify one or more additional active rauwolfia alkaloids resulted in isolation of rescinnamine, a compound having pharmacologic properties similar to those of reserpine, but producing less sedation, and less bradycardia in proportion to its hypotensive dose, than does reserpine.

Administration and Dosage

Rescinnamine is administered orally, in highly individualized dosages. Initially, 0.5 mg. twice daily for one week, with adjustment to 0.25 mg. once daily, for patients with anxiety states, and labile essential hypertension and tension.

General Clinical Uses

Clinical use has demonstrated that when rescinnamine is substituted for reserpine in the treatment of patients with hypertension, lassitude is much less pronounced;[116, 223] the complaint of somnolence is infrequent (in fact, a degree of insomnia has been the complaint of some patients). Patients who experience depression, sleepiness, diurnal lassitude and nightmares are thought likely to be more comfortable on rescinnamine, whereas patients more likely to benefit by sedation, prefer reserpine.[223] Most investigators agree that the rauwolfia alkaloids and rescinnamine exert their greatest therapeutic effect in the treatment of acute anxiety neurosis and tension states. The psychodynamic effect of rescinnamine on other types of neuroses is either very little, or none at all.

Specific Dermatological Uses

(See page 70.)

Toxic Effects and Side Reactions

Manifestations of reaction, reported to date, following therapy with rescinnamine, are:

Depression (mild) _____254
Dreams _____223
Drowsiness: lassitude: fatigability_____113, 254

These may occur especially during the first few days of therapy, but usually disappear, with continued use of the drug.

Diarrhea: looseness of stools: increased frequency of defecation _____113

Increased appetite: weight gain _____113

Nasal stuffiness to varying degree_____113, 254

This may be relieved by use of a vasoconstrictor topically and/or by internally-administered antihistamines.

Nervousness: insomnia _____223, 254

(Rescinnamine may increase gastric secretion: therefore, the drug must be used with caution in patients with a history of peptic ulcer.)

RECANESCINE
(*Harmonyl*—Abbott)

In 1955, Stoll and Hofmann reported the isolation of a new alkaloid from the root of Rauwolfia canescens Linn., which they named "canescine." This alkaloid has been investigated under the name of raunormine and, in addition, has been referred to as recanescine and deserpidine.[83]

The structural formula for recanescine (which is 11-desmethoxy-reserpine) is shown, following:

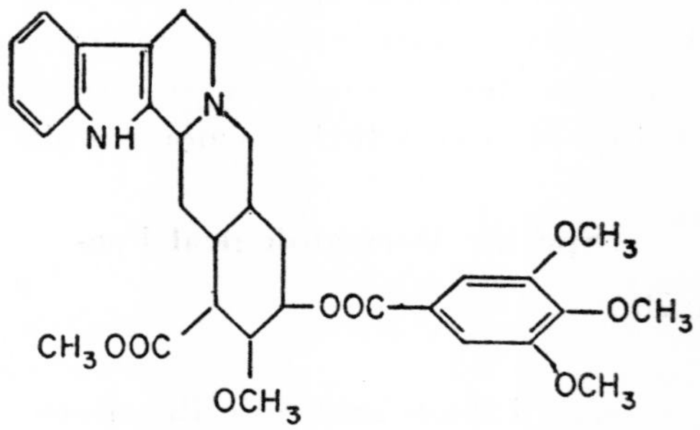

Pharmacologic Actions

Recanescine is a member of the same pharmacological group as reserpine and rescinnamine. Therefore, recanescine produces a mild, gradual and sustained lowering of blood pressure; a tranquilizing effect (usually without hypnosis); and a slowing of the heart rate.

Administration and Dosage

Recanescine is administered orally, for anxiety-tension states, in dosages of 0.25 mg., three or four times daily, with reduction of dosage after 10 days. For many patients with mild anxiety syndromes, the daily maintenance dosage is 0.25 mg.

General Clinical Uses

Recanescine is useful for its psychotherapeutic sedative action in mentally-disturbed patients, in conditions ranging from mild anxiety to major forms of mental illness: also for its antihypertensive action in patients with hypertensive disease.

Specific Dermatological Uses

(See page 70.)

Toxic Effects and Side Reactions

Dermal Reactions

Pruritus, generalized and severe, has required withdrawal of medication.[176]

*

Troublesome nasal congestion has been reported.[83, 176]

Central Nervous System Effects

"Recanescine seems to produce most of the side effects of various extracts of Rauwolfia serpentina, or of its main alkaloid, reserpine, and with comparable incidence."[176] Pepin and his associates[176] observed drowsiness and nightmares. Moyer et al.,[83] list the following side effects of recanescine, in descending order of frequency:

> Sedation
> Sense of well-being
> Weakness and fatigue
> Dizziness

Xerostomia

Dysuria

Gastrointestinal Disturbances

Increased appetite and weight gain..83, 176

Diarrhea 83

Constipation 83

According to Moyer *et al.*, "Recanescine appears to be less potent than comparable alkaloids and extracts of Rauwolfia serpentina; however, side reactions appear to be less annoying and somewhat less frequent."[163]

Specific Dermatological Uses of Rauwolfia— Alkaloids and Fractions

A recent report by the Robinsons[278] (Raymond, C. V., and Harry, Jr.) covering response by 2,087 patients with dermatoses reflecting changes in emotional reactions, included an evaluation of response by 600 patients, treated with various derivatives of rauwolfia (crude whole root; the alseroxylon fraction; and the alkaloids, reserpine, rescinnamine and recanescine). The conclusion of these investigators was:

"Annoying side effects in our series (nasal congestion, and the more serious profound depression) were encountered in more than 5% of patients treated. These derivatives are as useful in reducing anxiety as any of the drugs tested (sedatives, hydroxyzine hydrochloride, phenothiazines and meprobamate)—but the side effects made them unsuitable for use in patients with dermatoses."

The author and his associate have observed response of 538 private practice patients, to orally-administered rauwolfia, alkaloids and fractions, and in our experience, the incidence of side effects was even higher than that mentioned in the foregoing study. We have found, however, that rauwolfia and its derivatives are well suited to long-term dermatological therapy, for certain patients. The drugs are relatively inexpensive: once the patients' therapeutic levels are determined, repeated laboratory studies (with attendant expense) are unnecessary: and treatment can be continued for prolonged intervals, providing supervision is adequate.

Section III

Substituted Propanediols

SUBSTITUTED PROPANEDIOLS

Meprobamate   Miltown
                                     Equanil
Phenaglycodol   Ultran

MEPROBAMATE N.N.D.

(Miltown—Wallace Laboratories; *Equanil*—Wyeth Laboratories)

Meprobamate, or 2-methyl-2-n-propyl-1, 3-propanediol dicarbamate, was synthesized by Ludwig and Piech, in 1950. Structural formula for the compound is shown, following:

$$O \qquad CH_3 \qquad O$$
$$H_2N - C - OCH_2 - C - CH_2O - C - NH_2$$
$$CH_2CH_2CH_3$$

Meprobamate is the dicarbamate ester of a propanediol derivative, which is distinct from another propanediol derivative, mephenesin.

Pharmacologic Actions

The pharmacological and toxic actions of meprobamate were studied by Berger,[31, 32, 33, 261] utilizing rats, mice, dogs, cats, rabbits and monkeys. These studies indicated that meprobamate shares the central interneuronal blocking (skeletal muscle relaxant) action of mephenesin, but has an action of much longer duration. In man, the drug is more effective in reducing excessive proprioceptive muscle spasm than normal proprioceptive muscle tension. With little direct action on muscle itself, there is no alteration of the activity of the myoneural junction, and no conduction block in peripheral nerves. Meprobamate resembles barbiturates in that it has little effect on the autonomic nervous system. In this respect, the drug differs greatly from many other tranquilizers which have potent adrenolytic, atropine-like and antihistamine properties.[72] Meprobamate is rapidly absorbed through the gastrointestinal tract. After systemic absorption, the drug is apparently conjugated with glucuronic acid in the body, and excreted in the urine—about 10% being excreted unchanged. A simple test to determine meprobamate blood levels is not, at present, available. Although the over-all toxicity of the drug is low, it is capable of producing such a variety of side effects and untoward reactions, that indiscriminate use of the drug represents an unnecessary hazard to the patient.[166]

Administration and Dosage

Meprobamate is administered orally. (Parenteral use of the drug is now under investigative study.) The usual dosage for adults is 400 mg., two, three or four times daily. For insomnia, a single dose of 400 mg. or 800 mg. is recommended (to be taken upon retiring). For children, 3 years of age and older, the recommended initial dosage: 100 mg. to 200 mg., two or three times daily. For certain dermatological patients, the 200 mg. tablet permits flexible dosage schedules, and seems preferable to the 400 mg. tablet.[278]

General Clinical Uses

Available clinical evidence indicates that meprobamate may exert a useful calming effect in certain cases of abnormal motor activity seen in athetoid and dyskinetic patients; and is sometimes effective as an antispastic agent in fibrositis, where muscle spasm predominates.[166] Results have been poor in rheumatoid arthritis. Meprobamate exhibits anticonvulsant properties in experimental animals, but its value in epilepsy has not been clearly defined. On the basis of presently available clinical evidence, the drug appears to be useful as a mild hypnotic in simple insomnia, or as a psychotherapeutic agent, which can be employed in place of potent sedatives, and along with psychotherapy in the management of psychoneurotic anxiety and tension states. Meprobamate is useful as premedication in electroshock therapy, to allay preshock anxiety and postshock confusion and headache. Preliminary reports indicate that the drug may be useful in the treatment of alcoholism. Its value in paralysis agitans, and in the management of frank psychoses, has not yet been established.[166]

Specific Dermatological Uses

Meprobamate has been found to be of adjunctive value in the treatment of various dermatological conditions exacerbated by psychogenic factors. Selling[212, 213] reported that the drug cleared skin rashes of psychosomatic origin. LeVan and Wright,[144] in a study of 164 patients suffering from atopic and eczematoid dermatitis, neurodermatitis, psoriasis, lichen planus and chronic urticaria, reported that relaxation of nervous tension, diminution of anxiety and emotional stress and lessening of pruritus were more consistently observed, and were of greater degree than those obtained with reserpine therapy, in a previous study. The value of meprobamate in anogenital pruritus has been reported by Sokoloff;[226] and by Turrell:[238] in atopic dermatitis by Dixon;[69] and by Williamson:[252] in seborrheic dermatitis by Atkinson and Carpenter.[12]

Eisenberg[265] compared the effects of chlorpromazine, reserpine and meprobamate in 194 patients suffering from asthma, allergic headache, hay fever, eczema, gastrointestinal allergy, urticaria and angioneurotic edema. All exhibited persistent symptoms despite the usual allergy management, had complaints in excess of physical findings, or suffered from anxiety, tension or depression. While none of these patients recovered completely from allergic conditions, 38% showed definite improvement, as compared with 32% with chlorpromazine, and 21% with reserpine. Allergic headache and gastrointestinal allergy showed the greatest response, with 50% improvement: hay fever, 42% and asthma 41%. Favre,[78] also, reported on treatment of asthmatic patients with meprobamate.

Becker[29] reported study of response by 260 dermatological patients to meprobamate therapy. Most favorable results produced by administration of the drug (orally, in divided doses varying from 400 mg. to 2,400 mg. daily, occurred in cases of disseminated neurodermatitis, where there was an excellent-to-good effect, occurring in nearly 50% of all types of cases. Meprobamate, alone, however, was found to have little effect on pruritus, and required the addition of antipruritics, such as antihistamines or acetylsalicylic acid. In some cases of atopic eczema, excoriations were increased, and scratching appeared to be less inhibited. In Becker's experience, the incidence of allergic reactions was 4%: of undesirable side effects, 10%.

There have been other studies.[132, 262, 275]

Toxic Effects and Side Reactions

Allergic Phenomena - Dermal Reactions

As Becker reported, allergic reactions to meprobamate are generally of two types:

First: Urticaria and angioneurotic edema.—Such eruptions usually appeared within 48 hours of the initial dose of the drug, and disappeared in five to seven days after therapy was discontinued. Urticarial lesions were either localized, or generalized; pruritus might be intense, or non-existent.

Second: Morbilliform eruptions and toxic erythemata, typical of dermatitis medicamentosa.—These eruptions usually occurred after a week of therapy. In most instances, patients who experienced such reactions to meprobamate gave no history of allergy or previous drug intolerance, and there was no history of previous administration of mephenesin or similar compounds.

*

The following are interesting examples of reactions to meprobamate:

The report of McGee:[151]

"A 31-year-old female, a patient of mine, was given one tablet of Equanil, 400 mg., for relief of menstrual cramps. About an hour later, she developed mild to moderate generalized itching and skin rash. This was followed by generalized aching, chills and fever. I saw her about four hours after onset of the above, at which time she showed generalized erythematous maculopapular rash involving the entire body, extremities and face. Temperature 102° F. Physical examination otherwise negative. She was given Histadyl and Clopane capsules and epinephrine in oil by injection. The following morning she felt better but the rash persisted. That afternoon chills and fever recurred. Prednisone was administered orally with gradual clearing of symptoms during the next two days. There was considerable desquamation of skin following clearing of the rash. There was no history of skin rashes or allergy. She had had no unusual foods and had taken no medicaments during previous several weeks except prednisone, which she was taking on advice of a dermatologist for recurrent mouth ulcers. She had received no prednisone for some 36 hours preceding this reaction, and prednisone was used, as noted in treating the reaction with good results."

Kositchek[136] reported two reactions, both occurring within an hour after the first meprobamate tablet was taken, with both patients being incapacitated "and utterly miserable for a period lasting from three to seven days." All types of antihistamines were prescribed, but to no avail. The first patient responded, only after three days of treatment with steroids.

"Allergic Reaction to Meprobamate[5]

A 60-year-old white man, who had been in good health all his life, was started on treatment with meprobamate because of recent nervousness. About one hour after an initial dose of 400 mg., he noted numbness and tingling in his hands. He later went to sleep sitting in a chair but was awakened soon afterward by a severe shaking chill. When he was seen 15 minutes later, the chill was still present. His face was pallid, and there was a cyanosis of the nail beds. Temperature, heart, lungs and blood pressure were normal. The following day the skin of the entire body was markedly erythematous, having the appearance of skin severely burned by the sun. There was only slight cyanosis of the nail beds, but the hands were swollen. Temperature at this time was 100.2° F (39 C). There were no other abnormalities. In 24 hours the erythema was less severe, but swelling persisted in both hands, with numbness and tingling. There was no cyanosis of the nail beds, but the patient believed his legs were somewhat swollen. Temperature at this time was normal. There was a papular circumscribed eruption of 3 sq. cm. on each wrist."

Friedman and Marmelzat[97] reported seven cases of adverse reactions to meprobamate (only two of which are briefly reviewed, here). The third case described a 33-year-old female, without prior history of sensitivity or allergic disease, who took the drug, 400 mg. four times daily for 15 days. On the 16th day, she developed a small group of violaceous macules on the midback. Rapidly, within a period of two days, the eruption became generalized, with macules, papules and small vesicles. All of the lesions were purpuric in nature and showed tendency toward coalescence. The mucous membranes were not involved. The fourth case described a 49-year old female, with no history of drug sensitivity except development of a pruritic dermatosis two years previously, following systemic administration of penicillin. After the first dose of meprobamate, 800 mg., she developed an acute eruption involving the right breast, the axillae and back, and the entire inguinal area, in an acute process consisting of an erythematous base, with a loosely adherent furfuraceous scale. Lesions borders were not clearly demarcated, and diascopic pressure produced complete blanching of the erythema.

According to these investigators, skin lesions were interesting, in that the sites of predilection appeared to be the pelvic girdle, breast area, and the flexor surfaces of the arms. Less commonly involved were the trunk, anteriorly and posteriorly, and the legs. More remarkable was the fact that a patient who had never taken the compound before would develop the reaction within three to five hours after taking one tablet. Usually, in drug eruptions, the patient has had prior contact with the compound before developing dermatitis medicamentosa. In other words, prior sensitization is required before a reactive state is created, which on re-exposure gives clinical allergic response. A possible explanation of this phenomenon: these patients have been exposed in the past to chemically-related compounds, such as mephenesin.

*

There are other reports on this subject.[38, 59, 62, 77, 184, 212, 225]

*

Stroud[229] reported a generalized erythema, occurring eight days after the patient had taken a single tablet of meprobamate. The eruption was experimentally reproduced in the same patient, two months later. Another patient, who developed a diffuse erythema on two occasions, on the third, sustained, additionally, vasomotor collapse with loss of consciousness. Whenever such repeated reactions occurred, the initial ones were the mildest, eruptions tending to become more severe with every repetition of medication. It was Stroud's plea that there be early recognition of cutaneous eruptions, and discontinuance of therapy, in order to prevent more severe reactions.

*

Erythema multiforme[230] has been reported: exfoliative dermatitis[230] has been observed: and fixed drug eruptions,[206] following ingestion of meprobamate have been described. It is interesting to note that three of the latter were unilateral, and occurred on the hands.

*

Newman[167] reported the appearance of itching spots, which

appeared on the legs and forearms, of patients on meprobamate therapy. These spots became moist and scaly, and possessed every characteristic of nummular eczema. He stated: "Since this episode, I have carefully questioned my patients with nummular eczema for drug ingestion—and have been fortunate to elicit one additional nummular eczema-like eruption from meprobamate."

Purpuras

Gottlieb[104] was one of the first observers to report both reaction to meprobamate, and purpura, as a side effect of therapy.

A 42-year-old female with insomnia, tension headaches and anxiety neuroses was given meprobamate. After taking the third tablet she noted a feeling of warmth in her legs and thighs. Next day there was widespread hemorrhagic rash over axillae, breasts, chest, abdomen, arms, inner thighs and legs. She continued medication. Her temperature rose to 101° F. She had hard shaking chills and moderate edema of the legs and ankles. Three days later, the patient developed widespread purpura involving axillae, breasts, chest, arms, inner thighs and legs. Physical examination was otherwise unremarkable. The patient had a history of having taken no drugs or medicaments for the past six months.

Gottlieb supplied the hemogram, and added that he had heard of three similar cases, in all of which purpura appeared by the time the third tablet had been taken.

Carmel and Dannenberg[48] reported three cases of nonthrombocytopenic purpura in patients having no histories of allergy, purpura or drug sensitivity. All reactions occurred after from one to three meprobamate tablets had been taken for the first time. All three patients had positive capillary-fragility tests: negative blood counts: and in one patient, dramatic onset of eruption occurred a few hours after ingestion of the first tablet.

Witherspoon[255] reported a case of severe nonthrombocytopenic purpura accompanied by high fever and joint pains, following ingestion of seven tablets of meprobamate. He called attention to Gottlieb's report (of the patient who developed purpura hemorrhagica) wherein there was presence of purpura with fever, but clotting and bleeding times were prolonged, and he presented a case wherein both were normal, as was the platelet count. Witherspoon's patient displayed rapid regression of lesions, following therapy with corticotropin.

There are other reports concerning purpura.[62, 127, 132, 143] Epistaxis has been observed.[29] As is evident, meprobamate should not be prescribed for patients with known capillary fragility.[166]

*

In the study made by Klotz and Bernstein,[132] these reactions were observed following meprobamate therapy:

Dermatological manifestations _____73%
    Pruritus with, and without urticaria_____41%
    Exanthematic eruptions, morbilliform in type,
      usually involving trunk and lower extremi-
      ties _____37%
    Purpura simplex, with, and without
      thrombocytopenia _____22%
Systemic manifestations:
    A pattern of serum sickness, associated with fever ranging from 102° to 105° F., generally accompanied by skin manifestations and arthralgias, appeared in one-third of the cases studied. In several patients, bronchospasm occurred in those patients in whom fever and angioneurotic edema appeared, or were more severe.

*

There have been other reports of serum sickness:
    and bronchospasm _____49, 262

Cardiovascular Complications

Atrial flutter fibrillation arrhythmia (transient)_____132, 262
Dizziness: vertigo _____29, 174, 184
Hypotensive episodes_____211, 218
Syncope _____59, 184, 229

Central Nervous System Effects

Addiction: seizures_____138, 139, 184
    According to Essig and Ainslie: "These data show unequivocally that continued ingestion of large dosages of meprobamate can create physical dependence, manifested on abrupt withdrawal of the drug by hyper-irritability of the central nervous system and convulsions. The type of

addiction caused by meprobamate resembles that caused
by chronic intoxication with excessive amounts of barbiturates or alcohol" _____76
Drowsiness, sedation, somnolence _____29, 184, 225

These manifestations appear, to some observers, to be
an accompaniment of the mild somnifacient action of
meprobamate: by other observers, they are considered to
be side effects of therapy.

Euphoria _____132
Headache _____29
Inability to concentrate_____132
Muscular paralysis _____218, 278

According to Friedman and Marmelzat: "From the
pharmacology of the compound, muscular paralysis with
a large dose would appear to be a real possibility. For
ocular palsy to occur from two tablets (800 mg.) seems
impossible; yet it occurred in one patient." This patient
also experienced diplopia_____97
Paradoxical reactions with extreme excitement_____225

According to Friedman and Marmelzat: "After two
tablets in each instance, the meprobamate therapy was
discontinued. One tablet, subsequently, produced excitement and nervousness within one hour after oral administration" _____97
Toxicity due to overdosage and
and attempted suicide_____4, 29, 50, 57, 112, 147, 184, 218

Patients have exhibited alarming symptoms of coma,
shock, and in the most severe cases, complete vasomotor
collapse with respiratory failure.

Gastrointestinal Disturbances

Discomfort _____184
Hyperactivity _____97

According to Friedman and Marmelzat: "Intestinal
hyperactivity from therapy with a muscle-relaxing compound that is said to have no autonomic nervous system
effects seems rather paradoxical" . . . however . . . "we
have seen one case of intestinal hyperperistalsis, with rice
water stools."

Nausea and vomiting_____29, 225
Sluggishness of the small intestine_____225
Ulcer symptoms (one patient)_____225

The Robinsons observed response of 150 dermatological pations to meprobamate. The original dosage form was the 400 mg. scored tablet. After approximately 30 patients had been treated, it was found that the dose could be lowered without affecting the tranquilizing action appreciably; therefore, about one-half of the patients in this series received 200 mg. four times daily. Three patients developed scarlatiniform eruptions, which involuted quickly, following withdrawal of medication. An occasional patient complained that the muscular relaxation was annoying. In general, however, the drug was well tolerated and was effective in reducing emotional tension.

The author and his associate have observed response to therapy with meprobamate by more than 300 patients, with dermatoses complicated by psychogenic factors. In our experience, all patients who exhibited either objective or subjective improvement, initially, continued to be benefited by treatment with meprobamate. However, approximately one-fourth of our patients required increased dosage schedules, in order to maintain the beneficial effects which were observed initially, on a smaller dose. (We, too, favor use of the 200 mg. tablet.) We found that when patients are nonresponsive to the drug, increased dosages up to 1,600 mg. daily did not produce response.

We observed, as did Moyer and his associates,[275] that, as a rule, patients who respond to phenobarbital also respond to meprobamate. We could determine no significant difference between the degree of response to meprobamate and to phenobarbital, in patients responding to both drugs.

In general, our observations confirm the findings of Becker[29] and his associates. Meprobamate has little effect on pruritus, and requires concomitant administration of other antipruritic agents. We observed side effects, similar to those reported by Becker (with the exception of suicide, either attempted or accomplished), in a similar percentage of cases. We found meprobamate to be well-tolerated; however, close supervision of patients undergoing therapy with it is a prerequisite of treatment.

PHENAGLYCODOL N.N.D.

(*Ultran*—Eli Lilly & Company)

Phenaglycodol is 2-p-chlorophenyl-3-methyl-2, 3-butanediol, one of the synthetic diol compounds, for which the structural formula is:

$$Cl-\underset{}{\bigcirc}-\overset{\overset{OH}{|}}{\underset{\underset{CH_3}{|}}{C}}-\overset{\overset{OH}{|}}{\underset{\underset{CH_3}{|}}{C}}-CH_3$$

Pharmacologic Actions

Phenaglycodol has properties in common with the interneuronal blocking agents, such as mephenesin, and meprobamate, at least at the level of the spinal cord. Phenaglycodol and meprobamate have a common chemical derivation from mephenesin.[166]

In mice, cats and monkeys, phenaglycodol has a quieting effect, while producing minimal changes in blood pressure, respiration and electrocardiogram. In studies on selected reflex arcs, it has been shown to be a selective depressant of polysynaptic pathways, at the spinal and supraspinal level. After doses of phenaglycodol causing sedation but not sleep, in cats, the electroencephalogram shows a pattern of 9-12 c/sec. synchronous activity at both surface and deep electrodes.[222] The drug diminishes the severity of electrically-induced convulsions in animals. By rat-screening methods, phenaglycodol has both sedative and anticonvulsant properties.[108]

Administration and Dosage

Phenaglycodol is administered orally. The usual dose for adults: 300 mg., three or four times daily.

General Clinical Uses

From the standpoint of over-all clinical usefulness, phenaglycodol is probably most closely comparable to meprobamate: hence, it may be characterized as a mild sedative with weak muscle-relaxing properties. Phenaglycodol has been used to produce a calming, or ameliorating effect in patients with emotional instability, anxiety-tension states, and functional disorders. The drug may have usefulness in the adjunctive management of simple neuroses, but ultimate clinical usefulness must await the results of experience.[166] Evaluation in humans with difficult-to-control grand mal, petit mal or mixed epilepsy, also indicates that the drug has anticonvulsant activity.[108] Phenaglycodol lacks the structural characteristics which have been associated with anticonvulsant activity. In comparison with phenobarbital, larger doses are required; however, larger doses are also tolerated by humans, without excessive central nervous system depression.

Usually, drugs effective in grand mal are expected to increase the severity of petit mal, and vice versa. Since phenaglycodol is effective in petit mal, and the generalized seizures occurring in patients with focal brain damage, "it may prove advantageous in epilepsy of the mixed type."[108]

Phenaglycodol has been assayed, clinically, in the symptom-complex of geriatric agitation-tension states.[216] Study of 67 patients, ranging in ages from 60 to 94 years, has demonstrated that the drug is remarkably free from side effects. Repeated urinalyses, hemograms, renal and hepatic chemistries did not reveal a single instance of dysfunction after four to six months of continuous treatment. Two mild instances of drowsiness (not severe enough to preclude continuance of the drug), and one case of depression were the only untoward reactions. There was no impairment of alertness or mental acuity in those effectively tranquilized with phenaglycodol, which "is best suited for treatment of the mild to moderately severe levels of senile agitation."

Phenaglycodol has been evaluated in a group of (institutionalized) patients with tuberculosis.[18] The drug was found useful for relieving emotional tension and causing better acceptance of prolonged sanatorium care, involving medical and surgical antitubercular procedures.

The toxicity of phenaglycodol is low. No adverse effects on hepatic or hematopoietic function have been observed after long-term administration to animals or patients. In clinical experience, large doses are apparently without effect on blood pressure, pulse or respiration.[166]

Specific Dermatological Uses

A study of phenaglycodol as a tranquilizing agent for dermatological patients was made by Schwartz,[210] who administered the drug in a dosage range of 600 mg. to 900 mg. per 24-hour period, either singly, or in combination with local therapy, orally-administered antibiotics and steroids. The standard 300 mg. dose was prescribed on a twice-daily, or three-times-daily basis, depending upon the sedation required in each individual case. Eighty-one patients were included in his series, the largest groups of those having allergic eczematoid dermatitis and neurodermatitis. Excellent results were achieved in 34 patients: good results in 46 patients: and poor results in one patient. Schwartz observed that unlike meprobamate, patients on Ultran seldom experienced annoying or even incapacitating drowsiness. In the study reported by him, toxic manifestations were absent.

Toxic Effects and Side Reactions

Dermal Reactions

Cutaneous eruptions: rashes_____274
(In reports from 383 physicians, representing 6,806 patients, supplied by the Lilly Research Laboratories, dermatitis occurred in 0.4%)_____271

Central Nervous System Effects

Drowsiness: somnolence _____274
Inability to concentrate _____274
Paradoxical reactions with extreme excitement
and agitation _____274
(In reports, above-mentioned, drowsiness occurred in 2.3%; depression: anxiety occurred in 0.28%; headache occurred in 0.25%. Other side effects, which occurred in less than 0.15% of cases, included feelings of unreality, lethargy and insomnia.)_____271
(See reports by Moyer et al., page 86.)

Endocrine Imbalances

Gynecomastia _____271
(In reports, above-mentioned, included among "other

side effects," which occurred in less than 0.15% of cases, there is gynecomastia.)

Gastrointestinal Disturbances

Nausea, gastric distress and "disequilibrium"_____271
    (In reports, above-mentioned, these three gastrointestinal disturbances appeared, each, in 1% of cases.)

Moyer, Pevey and Kinross-Wright[274] reported on use of phenaglycodol in a series of psychotic patients, in two-thirds of whom response was satisfactory. Side effects were those observed with meprobamate: but the incidence was slightly higher for phenaglycodol (48%), than for meprobamate (30%).

Moyer, Pevey, Heider and Kinross-Wright[275] made a comparative study of four tranquilizing agents, phenobarbital and inert placebo, administered to 63 patients with nervousness, tension, anxiety, insomnia and various somatic disorders indicative of psychoneuroses. They found that with one exception, patients responsive to phenobarbital were uniformly responsive to phenaglycodol, while two patients nonresponsive to phenobarbital responded well to phenaglycodol. There was no apparent correlation between severity of disease, and responsiveness to either drug: also, no significant difference between degree of response to phenaglycodol, or phenobarbital in patients responding to both drugs. Patients, who presented evidence of depression prior to therapy, occasionally exhibited signs of increased depression or agitation following administration of phenaglycodol.

Section IV

Diphenylmethane Derivatives

DIPHENYLMETHANE DERIVATIVES

Benactyzine hydrochloride	Suavitil
Hydroxyzine hydrochloride	Atarax

BENACTYZINE HYDROCHLORIDE

(Suavitil—Merck Sharp & Dohme)

Benactyzine hydrochloride (Suavitil) is a member of that group of anticholinergic substances, several of which have selective activity upon various functions of the brain. This hydrochloride of the diethylaminoethyl ester of benzilic acid is represented by the following structural formula:

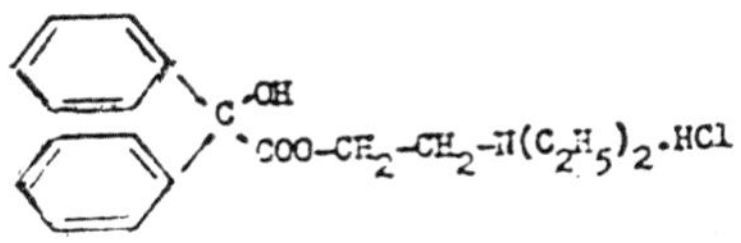

Pharmacologic Actions

Benactyzine hydrochloride, first prepared in Switzerland in 1936, has been recently studied by investigators in Scandinavia, Denmark, England and the United States.[3,15,52,63,103,110,131,191,250] Responses of laboratory animals (in which experimental neuroses were produced by various techniques), and of human subjects and patients, support the claim that benactyzine hydrochloride, in persons with, and without psychological disorders, reduces autonomic reaction to induced emotion, thereby producing a state of emotional and physical relaxation, without drowsiness. The drug raises the threshold for external stimuli, so that the patient, in a state of tension, arising from excessive strain, no longer reacts to stimuli, which previously would have provoked irritation. He feels as though a "barrier had been interposed between himself and his problems," of which he is aware, but which no longer distress and confuse him. When given in therapeutic dosages, the drug is eliminated from the body within a few hours; is apt to produce no euphoria (although this side effect has been mentioned); and to date, no withdrawal symptoms have been detected.

Benactyzine hydrochloride has specific central nervous system action, differing from that produced by other drugs, to date. The peripheral parasympatholytic effects[275] include: antispasmodic action on the gastrointestinal tract; inhibition of salivary secretions; and pupillary dilatation, one-tenth that of atropine in equal doses. Although benactyzine hydrochloride is not as versatile as chlorpromazine, having slight or no effect on body temperature, and no adrenolytic effects, it does possess low antihistaminic properties, a quinidine-like action on the heart three times as potent as that of quinidine, and local anesthetic action almost equal to that of codeine. In contrast to chlorpromazine and reserpine, it has a pronounced effect on the human electrocardiogram,[275] reducing the normal rhythm with partial to complete blocking of the alpha waves; however, other waves, including dysrhythmias are unaffected.

Considering that synapses in the central nervous system have acetylcholine as a chemical transmitter, it is conceivable that benactyzine acts by virtue of its anticholinergic properties. However, thus far nothing is known about mode of action, or specific anatomic or functional parts of the central nervous system upon which the drug produces effects. In the opinion of certain investigators,[275] benactyzine hydrochloride exhibits rather diffuse action on the pathways connecting the cortex, thalamus and other subcortical structures, and the spinal cord. As an anticholinergic, benactyzine hydrochloride appears to be about twenty times more potent than chlorpromazine, but a relatively poor histamine antagonist, being ten times less active than chlorpromazine, and twenty times less active than diphenhydramine (Benadryl).

In relatively high doses, benactyzine hydrochloride causes hyperexcitability and clonic convulsions in animals. No taming effect has been observed. Hexobarbital (Evipal) anesthesia was markedly prolonged; the effects of acetylcholine on the isolated gut, and blood pressure were diminished; and the action of epinephrine on blood pressure was enhanced by this compound.[250]

Administration and Dosage

The drug is administered orally, as (scored) tablets, each containing 1 mg. of the active ingredient. The usual dosage for adults: 1 mg. three times daily for two or three days. Then, dosage may be gradually increased to 3 mg. three times daily, if favorable results are not manifest. When beneficial results are obtained, however, they are usually evident within one or two weeks.

General Clinical Uses

Benactyzine hydrochloride has been recommended for the relief of tension and anxiety in psychotic and nonpsychotic patients.[3] The drug reduces the psychic pain, fear, and resulting inhibitory avoidance responses engendered by stress. It is known that benactyzine hydrochloride facilitates the orienting response and the formation of new conditioned reflexes, thus counteracting the inhibitory state of the higher cortical activity. The drug has proved itself to be mildly antidepressant and particularly effective in relieving the ruminative-obsessive aspects of the depressive mood. However, it has failed to relieve the sleep disturbance of the depressed patient, and often brought to the fore, anxious tension. The antidepresseant effect of the drug appears to be thus due to strengthening the ego boundaries rather than to diminution of excitability. Benactyzine hydrochloride, when combined with meprobamate has been recommended for the treatment of depression, as a step which allows patients to recover, thus screening and reducing the number of patients requiring electroshock therapy.[3]

To summarize: benactyzine hydrochloride appears to be particularly effective in psychoneuroses with anxiety reaction, but can be effective, also, in psychoneuroses with depressive and obsessive compulsive reactions, and perhaps, in compulsive alcoholism.

Specific Dermatological Uses

Observation of response by patients with various dermatological disorders, to whom benactyzine hydrochloride was administered alone, and in combination with other therapeutic agents, has been reported by the author and his associate.[250] Diagnoses of patients so treated, were:

Diagnosis	Number of Patients Males	Females
Acne rosacea	--	2
Angioneurotic edema and urticaria	1	--
Atopic dermatitis	4	4
Chronic infectious eczematoid dermatitis	2	2
Dermatitis medicamentosa (reserpine)	--	1
Glossodynia	--	1

Lupus erythematosus, subacute, disseminated ____ __ 1
Neurodermatitis _____ __ 1
Psoriasis _____ __ 3
Seborrheic dermatitis _____ __ 1
      Total_____ 7 16

In this series of 23 patients, one patient failed to return, and inquiry regarding his status elicited no response. Comments, therefore, cover responses by 22 patients. All were drawn from private practice, and were, by their own admissions, tense, plagued with anxiety, prone to preoccupation and rumination. All but two of these patients had had previous therapy with other tranquilizers. The drug was administered in the form of 1 mg. tablets, to be taken once, twice, three or four times daily as conditions warranted. All patients were observed at weekly intervals. At first, patients were instructed to take the medication before retiring, or midmorning, midafternoon and midevening, but after reports of gastric distress, patients were instructed to take the medication immediately after a meal.

Side effects, encountered singly, or in combination, in this series were:

	Number of Patients	
	Males	Females
Memory loss	__	2
Fainting	__	1
"Unable to speak"	__	1
Dizziness	__	3
Drowsiness, lethargy, "tired all the time," "just want to sit," "hangover"	2	5
Apathy or general detachment	1	4
Nausea, vomiting, heartburn, bloating	__	5
Increased appetite, with consequent weight gain	__	2
"Weak in the legs," "legs feel like rubber"	__	3
"Can't move my legs—I have been paralyzed"	__	1
General weakness	__	3
Manifestations of reaction termed "allergic responses"	1	1
Vague uneasiness—"something is the matter—I don't know what"—with consequent increase in anxiety and tension	6	12

Responses of 22 patients to benactyzine hydrochloride were:

	Number of Patients	
	Males	Females
Tolerated benactyzine hydrochloride, and showed not only lessening of tension, but also dermatological improvement	1	3
Tolerated the drug, but showed marked dermatological exacerbation	5	6
Tolerated the drug, and maintained dermatological status quo	1	3
Serious side effects	--	3

The serious side effects manifested by three patients were:
—fainting, inability to speak, hypotension
—memory loss
—inability to move legs, with consequent fear of having had a stroke

Among the patients who experienced not-so-serious side effects, the following were observed:

A male patient, who had been taking meprobamate three times daily for several months, took benactyzine hydrochloride 1 mg. three times daily for two weeks. He asked to be put back on the "old pills—because the new ones do nothing for me. I can't sleep. I'm all jittery."

A female patient, aged 34 years, who had been under observation and therapy for 15 years, and whose menstrual cycles were known to be regular, experienced delay in ovulation and menstruation when benactyzine therapy was instituted a couple of days prior to expected date of ovulation. It was postulated by us, that benactyzine hydrochloride may have some modifying effect upon the menstrual cycle, as is the case with chlorpromazine, perphenazine, trimeprazine (in our experience), and reserpine.

Worsening of various dermatoses in 18 patients under benactyzine therapy was attributed to mental stress induced by the feeling of "something wrong."

Derivatives of rauwolfia serpentina, steroid hormones and antihistamines were found to manifest no incompatibilities when administered concomitantly with benactyzine hydrochloride.

Results of this study did not confirm the observations of others that patients on a dosage of benactyzine hydrochloride 1 mg. three times daily experienced no side effects, although we conceded that the drug was administered to a group of hypersensitive individuals. Our conclusions:

"We do not feel that benactyzine hydrochloride is an agent suitable for indiscriminate use in dermatologic practice. We concur with other investigators that side effects, although transient, appear to be a disadvantage in the possible regular use of this drug in patients of known, or suspected sensitivities."

The following opinion has been expressed regarding the foregoing:[245]

"Dr. Ashton Welsh and Dr. Mitchell Ede reported recently on another drug to relieve emotional tension in dermatoses, namely benactyzine hydrochloride, an anticholinergic agent marketed under the name of Suavitil. It was pointed out, and I agree completely, that this preparation has extremely undesirable side effects, making it useless in dermatology."

Toxic Effects and Side Reactions

Dermal Reactions

Maculopapular eruption _____131
Rash _____275

Allergic Phenomena

(See page 92.)

Cardiovascular Complications

Hypotension _____250
Palpitations and "throbbing" sensations_____3, 52, 63, 131, 275
Tachycardia _____15
(See page 92.)

Central Nervous System Effects

Anxiety _____15, 172, 191, 250
Apathy, general detachment, lassitude:
    feelings of depersonalization _____15, 52, 63, 250
Clumsiness: ataxia_____15, 52, 191, 250, 275
Depression: compulsion_____172
Dizziness: vertigo _____3, 15, 52, 63, 110, 191, 250, 275
Drowsiness _____172, 191, 250
Dryness of the mouth_____15, 52, 63, 131, 172, 191, 250, 275

EEG changes, in normal subjects, with striking
  suppression of normal rhythm _____52, 191
Euphoria: "couldn't care less"—
  "slap-happy" _____52, 131, 172, 191, 275
Inappropriate behavior _____275
Muscular relaxation: altered sensation in limbs:
  some gait impairment _____15, 52, 191, 250, 275
Perceptive changes:
  Difficulty in reading fine print:
    blurring of vision _____52, 110, 191
  Micropsia _____52
  Nystagmus _____275
  Pupillary dilatation _____3, 15, 131, 275
Restlessness _____15, 250
Thought-blocking: loss of memory:
  inability to concentrate _____15, 52, 63, 131, 172, 191, 250, 275

Endocrine Imbalances

Modification of menstrual cycle _____250
Psychosexual disorders, particularly in women, must be ap-
  proached with care. The formation of overt homosexual
  relationships, without feelings of shame, following benactyzine hydrochloride therapy, has been reported _____63

Gastrointestinal Disturbances

Diarrhea _____191
Gastric distress: nausea: vomiting _____15, 52
  usually associated with nystagmus _____275

*

The incidence of side effects is high—ranging from 40% to
60% in various studies, when benactyzine hydrochloride is given
in average doses of 2 mg. three times daily (which are necessary to
elicit improvement). Patients taking as much as 4 mg. three times
daily invariably experience objectionable side effects.[275]

HYDROXYZINE HYDROCHLORIDE N.N.D.
*(Atarax—*J. B. Roerig & Company)

Hydroxyzine hydrochloride (Atarax) is 1-(p-Chlorobenzhy-
dryl)-4-[2-(2-hydroxyethoxy)ethyl] piperazine dihydrochloride, the
structural formula of which may be represented as follows:

$$Cl - \bigcirc \bigcirc \quad HC - N \Big\langle \begin{array}{c} CH_2 - CH_2 \\ \\ CH_2 - CH_2 \end{array} \Big\rangle N - CH_2 \cdot CH_2 \cdot O \cdot CH_2 \cdot CH_2 OH \cdot 2HCl$$

Hydroxyzine

Pharmacologic Actions

Hydroxyzine hydrochloride, which is similar in chemical structure and pharmacological action to some of the antihistamines, produces depression of the central nervous system.[166] Sedation is the most prominent action of hydroxyzine hydrochloride, and forms the basis for its clinical use. The drug also appears to exert some actions similar to those of chlorpromazine; however, these are not sharply enough defined to permit pharmacological classification as a chlorpromazine-like drug. Hydroxyzine is a slightly neurotropic, but definitely myotropic antispasmodic agent, a hypotensive agent, and an anesthetic.[122]

Guinea-pigs injected intravenously with 2.5 mg. of hydroxyzine per kilo of body weight are protected against over 800 lethal doses of histamine; the reduction of spasm induced by acetylcholine in the ileum of the guinea-pig indicates that the antispasmodic action of the drug is similar to that of atropine. The action of hydroxyzine on spasm induced by barium chloride in the jejunum of rabbits is equivalent to 80% that of papaverine. In dogs, an injection of hydroxyzine produces a transient drop in arterial blood pressure, which is lowered by about 40% as compared with the initial level. The rhythm and amplitude of respiration are increased.[121]

Local anesthetic action is manifested in the following: as compared with novocain, the potency of hydroxyzine amounts to 316%, as a contact anesthetic (test on the cornea of guinea-pigs) and to 200% as a conduction anesthetic. As for systemic anesthetic action, hydroxyzine is neither a ganglio-plegic agent nor a curarimimetic drug; it does not induce any lipothymia, even when large doses are administered.

Hydroxyzine acts centrally, but is not hypnogenic. It also possesses anticonvulsant action, but does not prevent convulsions, following administration of convulsive agents: however, in animals, it prolongs survival time. (Barbiturates prevent crises and death by convulsive agents.) Hydroxyzine prevents the trembling effect produced by nicotine in rabbits, induces hypothermic effect, acting through the heat-regulating center, neutralizes the emetic effect of apomorphine, and has analgesic effect.

The foregoing pharmacological data are important, because they explain the wide range of possibilities offered by the drug.

Administration and Dosage

Hydroxyzine hydrochloride is administered orally and parenterally, in highly-individualized dosages. For adults, the usual oral dosage is one 25 mg. tablet taken three or four times daily. For children three to six years: one 10 mg. tablet or one teaspoon Atarax Syrup (2 mg./cc.) three times daily; for children over six years: two 10 mg. tablets, or two teaspoons of Atarax Syrup three times daily. Hydroxyzine hydrochloride may be administered intramuscularly, as Atarax Parenteral Solution (25 mg./cc.), the dosage to be dependent upon the requirements. Usually: 25 mg. to 50 mg. (1 cc. to 2 cc.) intramuscularly, repeated every four hours, as required. Proportionately lower dosages for children.

General Clinical Uses

Hydroxyzine hydrochloride has been found effective, as a tranquilizing agent, in various types of organic or functional disturbances;[56] psychoneuroses;[61] tension states;[215, 260] syndromic psychoneurotic amebiasis;[214] functional or non-organic hypertension (but the drug is ineffective in hypertensive disease); prior to certain procedures such as bronchoscopy; for the treatment of cardiac arrhythmias; for tranquilization in gynecologic procedures, and obstetrics.

The outstanding characteristic of hydroxyzine appears to be its ability to muffle exaggerated responses to external or internal stimuli, without dulling the patient's perspective or sense of values. In this regard, the drug is considered distinctly superior to tranquilizing agents which induce hypnosis on the one hand, and those producing euphoria, on the other.

Hydroxyzine is valuable for anxious children; and for hyper-kinetic children in whom drug-induced psychic impairment would be undesirable.

Specific Dermatological Uses

There have been several reports on use of hydroxyzine in dermatological therapy.[195, 196, 278] The Robinsons and their associate[195] reported on administration of the drug to 159 patients, with the following diagnoses:

> atopic dermatitis (extensive)
> neurodermatitis (localized)
> factitious dermatitis
> psoriasis
> dermatitis herpetiformis
> lichen planus
> nummular eczema
> dyshidrosis
> alopecia areata
> pruritus ani or pruritus vulvae
> urticaria
> seborrheic dermatitis
> rosacea

The usual dosage was 10 mg. to 25 mg., four times daily. Ataraxic effect was satisfactory in 132 patients, who stated that they experienced some degree of release from previously existing tension. The calming effect was most pronounced in patients with atopic dermatitis, neurodermatitis, factitious dermatitis, lichen planus, pruritus ani or pruritus vulvae, and urticaria. Statements made by 15 patients indicated that in these persons the tranquilizing effect was only fair, and in 12 patients, hydroxyzine therapy was ineffectual.

Seven patients reported drowsiness, which disappeared after two or three days of continued medication. Two patients noted persistent sleepiness. Four patients who had received the drug for one week complained of dryness of the oropharynx, but this symptom was not severe enough to require cessation of therapy. The first four patients complained of a "fluttering feeling in the stomach," but when the medicament was taken after meals, symptoms subsided. Pruritus was noted by one patient who had been taking hydroxyzine for two weeks, and it became necessary to discontinue administration of the drug and substitute another compound. One patient developed severe headache, after taking the drug for one week, but when administration of hydroxyzine was discontinued and phenobarbital (15 mg. four times a day) substituted, the headaches disappeared. Upon administration of placebo tablets, the patient did not develop headaches, but when hydroxyzine was readministered, the headaches recurred.

Objective evaluation in 41 selected patients led to the conclusion that hydroxyzine hydrochloride is valuable adjunctive therapy in the treatment of patients with dermatoses in which emotional tension is a factor. Comparative studies based on subjective evidence led to the conclusion that hydroxyzine hydrochloride produced as satisfactory an ataraxic effect as other tranquilizers presently available.

Another report by the same investigators,[196] described the use of hydroxyzine hydrochloride in the treatment of 300 dermatological patients: and still another report[278] described use of the drug in the treatment of 479 patients with various dermatoses, in which emotional stress was thought to be a productive or aggravating factor. Diagnoses of patients were the same as those mentioned in the earlier study.[195] Subjective evaluation, based on patients' statements, led to the conclusion that the ataractic effect of the drug was satisfactory in 378 patients. Objective evaluation in 140 patients led to the conclusion that the use of hydroxyzine hydrochloride is valuable adjunctive therapy in the treatment of patients with dermatoses in which emotional tension was a factor. Adverse reactions were minimal. Mild lethargy was commonly observed after initiation of treatment with hydroxyzine hydrochloride, but this symptom disappeared after two or three days of continued medication. Dryness of the oropharynx was observed in 14 patients: one had slight pruritus; two developed headache; and one complained of severe vertigo. Comparative studies with other drugs led to the conclusion that hydroxyzine hydrochloride produced as satisfactory an ataractic effect as other tranquilizers and sedatives presently available.

Seneca[214] studied a series of eight patients with amebiasis, where the main manifestations were psychoneurosis. Specific anti-amebic treatment consisted of antibiotics: and symptomatic treatment of psychoneuroses included use of hydroxyzine hydrochloride, in doses ranging from 10 mg. to 25 mg. four times daily, until symptoms were controlled. The only side effects encountered with hydroxyzine hydrochloride were sleepiness, drowsiness and mild headache. All patients tolerated the drug very well.

Toxic Effects and Side Reactions

Dermal Reactions - Allergic Phenomena

Pruritus_____195, 196, 271, 274
    Severe enough to warrant cessation of therapy_____195
Rhinorrhea _____271, 274
Urticaria _____278

Central Nervous System Effects

Drowsiness_____195, 196, 240, 271, 278
    This usually appears, initially, and subsides after two
    or three days. However, occasionally it is persistent.
Dryness of the mouth and throat_____ 195, 196, 271, 274, 278
Headache_____195, 196, 274, 278
    (See page 99.)
Muscular weakness: unsteadiness _____195, 196, 271
Vertigo _____196

Gastrointestinal Disturbances

Increased intestinal peristalsis _____271, 274
Weight gain _____271, 274

Section V

Ureides and Amides

UREIDES AND AMIDES

Ectylurea

Oxanamide

Nostyn

Quiactin

ECTYLUREA

(Nostyn—Ames Company, Inc.)

Ectylurea (Nostyn) is the higher melting isomer of 2-ethylcrotonylurea, an unsaturated open-chain ureide, having the following structural formula:

$$CH_3CH_2-\underset{\underset{H\text{-}C\text{-}CH_3}{\overset{||}{}}}{\overset{\overset{O}{\overset{||}{}}}{C}}-\overset{\overset{O}{\overset{||}{}}}{C}\ NH\ \overset{\overset{O}{\overset{||}{}}}{C}\ NH_2$$

The compound is almost insoluble in water, yet, when administered orally, its effects are manifested within 15 minutes.

Pharmacologic Actions

The main pharmacologic interest in ectylurea lies in its low toxicity and the wide range of dosage, which can be used to induce sedation without incurring side effects.[181] Ectylurea is rapidly absorbed and metabolized and has no effect on the hematopoietic, hepatic, respiratory, temperature-regulating or renal systems: or, on the nonprotein nitrogen, or blood sugar. It does not cause hangover, or grogginess, and there is no evidence of habituation or withdrawal symptoms.[86] Ectylurea produces mild depression of the central nervous system, an action which it shares with other substituted urea compounds. In experimental animals, it exerts sedative effects from doses much lower than those required to produce hypnosis.[73]

Administration and Dosage

Ectylurea is administered orally. The optimal dosage has not been firmly established: amounts ranging from 0.15 Gm. to 0.3 Gm., three or four times daily may be employed, apparently without appreciable risk of toxicity.[73]

General Clinical Uses

Ectylurea has been employed as a mild neurosedative, or calming agent in the treatment of simple anxiety and nervous tension, and its tension-relieving effects have been reported in adults of all age groups;[85] and in hyperexcitable children, with behavior problems. It is not a hypnotic per se, but may promote sleep in some patients whose tension and anxiety are responsible for insomnia. There is no evidence that the drug is of any benefit in alcoholic patients, or those with frank psychoses.

Ferguson[84] has found that ectylurea, in a dosage range of 50 mg. to 150 mg., three times daily, induced over-all calmness, which made the patient easier to manage, and more capable of participating in activities. This was especially true of elderly patients, who needed mild medication for anxiety and tension states, without the sedative or habit-forming properties of the barbiturates.

A recent study by Bauer and his associates,[28] on 172 patients with tension, anxiety or insomnia, when ectylurea was administered in unit doses ranging from 150 mg. to 900 mg., and in total daily doses varying from 150 mg. to 1,200 mg., confirmed the fact that the drug is mild, non-habit forming, tranquilizing, of low toxicity, induces daytime sedation without mental depression, and promotes sleep by the alleviation of tension and anxiety. The sedative, as well as soporific action of the drug was demonstrated in patients with glandular conditions, such as hyperthyroidism, or the climacteric.

Twenty-two of the 172 patients developed side effects, and eight of these refused further treatment because of them. Side effects were:

> dizziness
> nervousness
> chest pains
> headache
> marked daytime drowsiness
> anorexia
> urinary dribbling or frequency
> dryness of the mouth
> metallic taste in the mouth

These investigators reported that in view of the smallness of the doses, it was doubtful that the nervousness and chest pains, observed in three patients at a daily dosage level of 450 mg., were actually due to the drug, for they were never observed at any higher dose, nor did these patients continue to complain of them after the drug had been continued for several days. However, they are recorded in order that physicians might be on the alert for such possibility, in the further evaluation of the drug.

It was considered questionable whether daytime sleepiness should be looked upon as a side effect, although this effect seems to be germane to the true action of ectylurea. It should be kept in mind that tension and anxiety may mask a state of fatigue, symptoms of which include drowsiness, and the symptom of sleepiness may appear upon the relief of tension and anxiety. If the seven patients who reported sleepiness, and the three patients who reported nervousness and chest pains are excluded, then there were 12 individuals who manifested untoward effect. Clinically, these effects were similar to those produced by imbalance of the autonomic nervous system, and may have been due to some underlying condition, since there is pharmacologic evidence that in laboratory animals, approximately 80% of the LD_{50} dose intraperitoneally of ectylurea is required to affect the vagal nuclei.

In certain pediatric cases,[10] daily administration of ectylurea has resulted in diminution of restlessness and irritability. A clinical study of the effects of the drug on hyperexcitable, uncooperative, or anti-social behavior patterns of 51 children, aged two to 12 years, who were difficult to manage in a hospital, has been reported with fairly detailed results, including effects after the drug was stopped; effect on enuresis; response of patients with postmeningitis behavior problems; and patients requiring minor operative procedures; effect of increased dosage; and influence on weight. The drug effectively normalized 35 patients; was of minimal or questionable value in eight; of no value in four; and adversely affected the behavior in four. No toxic effects were seen.

Previously, the same authors[9] studied the effects of ectylurea in nine children, who were mute, deaf, mentally retarded, or presented behavior problems following recovery from tuberculous meningitis. A case history is presented for each patient. The drug had a relaxing effect on hyperactivity, spasticity, and insomnia. In some cases, improvement was maintained after the drug was stopped, but in most cases, symptoms recurred.

Specific Dermatological Uses

To the author's knowledge, therapy with ectylurea in dermatological conditions, has not been reported.

Toxic Effects and Side Reactions

Dermal Reactions

Cutaneous eruptions: rash—

"In clinical studies, the only side effect encountered to date has been a skin rash, which appears in considerably less than 1% of patients"..73

In a study reported by Ferguson and Linn "when 525 patients, ranging in ages from 17 to 25 years, were treated with Nostyn in dosages ranging from 60 mg. to 300 mg. three or four times daily for as long as six months), in 2%, or nine patients, occasional side effects consisted of rash. . . . "...86

Central Nervous System Effects

Dizziness 28, 86
Drowsiness 28, 86
Headache 28
Nervousness 28
Urinary dribbling or frequency 28
Xerostomia: metallic taste 28

Gastrointestinal Disturbances

Anorexia 28
Nausea 86

OXANAMIDE

(*Quiactin*—The Wm. S. Merrell Company)

Oxanamide (Quiactin) is a new quieting agent, unrelated, structurally, to many of the psychotherapeutic drugs in clinical use, today. Chemically, the drug is 2-ethyl-3-propylglycidamide, the structural formula for which appears, following:

$$CH_3 - CH_2 - CH_2 - \overset{\displaystyle H}{\underset{\displaystyle \diagdown O \diagup}{C}} - \overset{\displaystyle C_2H_5}{\underset{\displaystyle \diagup}{C}} - \overset{\displaystyle O}{\underset{\displaystyle \parallel}{C}} \, NH_2$$

Quiactin occurs as a tasteless, white, crystalline solid, with little or no odor. One part is soluble in 95 parts of water at 30° C. Clinical acceptance of the tablet has been excellent.

Pharmacologic Actions

Oxanamide has a central depressant action, in animals, generally resembling that of the short-acting barbiturates (secobarbital, pentobarbital, and the like). Its milligram potency, as determined in animals, is roughly one-fifth to one-eleventh that of pentobarbital; one-fourth that of ethylisoamylbarbituric acid; and similar to that of a-monobromoisovaleryl-urea: its duration of action is similar to these hypnotics, and its margin of safety, at least as large. Repeated daily administration of comparatively high doses of Quiactin are nontoxic and noncumulative in laboratory animals.[244] These properties are of extreme clinical significance. Approximately 90% of the drug is conjugated or metabolized in the body; animal studies show urinary, but no fecal excretion of the drug, and there has been no indication that it may be irritating to the gastric mucosa.

Administration and Dosage

Individual patient-requirements determine the dosage for Quiactin. (This is generally accepted, now, for all mood-influencing drugs.) For quieting action, one Quiactin 400 mg. tablet, given three or four times daily, is the usual dosage. For insomnia, two 400 mg. tablets of Quiactin given at bedtime, or as required.

General Clinical Uses

Oxanamide has been studied in insomnia, anxiety states and psychotic excitement. Feuss and Gragg[88] studied a group of "chronically irritated" institutionalized females. Quarreling was reduced; patients continued to work efficiently, and slept soundly at night. The drug was found to be of low toxicity, pleasant to the taste, and seemed "to improve the behavior of irritable patients to an extent that connot be explained by chance."

Coats and Gray[54] treated a group of 30 hospitalized patients (ranging in age from 26 to 79 years) with a wide variety of psychopathologic disorders, in a daily dosage of 1.6 Gm., orally. None had responded to previous therapy. Improved behavior was noted with respect to anxiety, tension, hostility, mood and socialization. There were no side effects during treatment, or withdrawal effects at the end of the treatment period. Laboratory studies conducted in all patients before, during, and after treatment demonstrated no impairment of function of the vital organs.

Proctor[187] administered Quiactin to 40 patients (at a hosiery mill), who had complained of psychomotor activity, agitation, restlessness and tension headaches. According to him "the drug has an action similar to meprobamate, but it seems . . . that its activity is more prolonged and its sedative effect is not quite so marked, while the tranquilizing effect is greater."

Feuss and Ivanov[89] treated 30 female out-patients, who were chosen, regardless of diagnosis, age or length of illness, but who were having undue difficulty in making a satisfactory adjustment socially, as manifested by persistent distressing anxiety, apathy and over-irritability. All had previously been given chlorpromazine, reserpine, meprobamate, promazine or combinations of these. These drugs were discontinued. Quiactin was given in dosages varying from 1.2 to 3.6 Gm. daily, in three divided doses; and the dosage for each patient was not changed during the 2-months' period of study. None of the patients complained of subjective symptoms from Quiactin, and its freedom from toxicity and unpleasant subjective symptoms, as well as its apparent effectiveness in aiding these patients to control their anxiety, enabled them to resume progress toward social readjustment, whereas the unpleasant subjective symptoms of some of the other psychotherapeutic drugs slowed down, or arrested this program.

Quiactin is a normalizer, a quieting agent for overly-anxious patients; it improves the behavior in the irritable, quarrelsome person, calms the restless, tense person; and allows easier social readjustment. In the dosages recommended by the manufacturer, it rarely produces drowsiness.

Specific Dermatological Uses

Study of oxanamide, as a tranquilizing agent was undertaken by the author and his associate, during January, 1958, and has been pursued without interruption, for six months. The following constitutes a preliminary report of our observations regarding the efficacy of this agent in 460 patients, having some strong emotional factor either as a cause of dermatitis, or as a result of it.

All patients were drawn from private practice; all were observed at weekly intervals, and only those who faithfully followed prescribed therapeutic regimens are included in this report. Oxanamide was the sole internal therapeutic agent administered for tranquilizing effect, during the study period; topical therapeutic regimens were varied as conditions required; actinic therapy was administered when, and as indicated. The history of each patient was carefully scrutinized for past medication with tranquilizing agents, administered by us, or prescribed by others. Pertinent data, such as normal hemograms, urinalyses, blood pressures and pulse rates were recorded for comparative purposes.

Patients were divided into two groups: those having had, and those having never had previous therapy with tranquilizing agents. The following tables show number of patients, age groups, dosage schedules and diagnoses:

PATIENTS HAVING HAD THERAPY WITH OTHER TRANQUILIZING AGENTS

(Including phenothiazines; rauwolfia, alkaloids and fractions; substituted propane-diols; diphenylmethane derivatives, transferred to oxanamide therapy)

Diagnoses	Oxanamide 400 mg. twice daily		Oxanamide 400 mg. three times daily		Oxanamide 400 mg. four times daily	
	Females Ages 16-69	Males Ages 18-72	Females Ages 17-64	Males Ages 19-57	Females Ages 19-49	Males Ages 23-51
Acne: indurata	6	4	2	1	1	1
rosacea	8	2	3	1	--	--
vulgaris	6	1	4	2	1	--
Angioneurotic edema: urticaria	2	1	2	1	3	1
Atopic dermatitis	8	5	4	1	2	--
Chronic infectious eczema-toid dermatitis	14	6	5	2	1	1
Contact dermatitis	16	7	6	3	--	--
Dermatitis medicamentosa	2	1	2	1	--	--
Hyperhidrosis	6	2	4	2	1	--
Intertrigo	3	--	4	--	--	--
Lichen planus	3	1	3	--	--	--
Lichen sclerosus et atrophicus	3	--	2	--	--	--
Lupus erythematosus: subacute disseminated	4	--	2	--	--	--

chronic discoid	2	..	1	..	..	..
Lymphocytoma	..	..	..	..	..	1
Miliaria	6	..	3	..	..	..
Neurodermatitis	11	4	5	1	..	..
Pruritus ani et vulvae	9	6	3	1	..	..
Psoriasis	6	4	5	1	..	..
Raynaud's disease	1	..	1	..	..	..
Seborrheic dermatitis	6	2	3	1	..	..
Stasis dermatitis	9	4	2	1	..	..
Totals	131	50	66	19	9	4

Grand Total...............279

PATIENTS NEVER HAVING HAD THERAPY WITH OTHER TRANQUILIZING AGENTS

Diagnoses	Oxanamide 400 mg. twice daily		Oxanamide 400 mg. three times daily		Oxanamide 400 mg. four times daily	
	Females Ages 16-47	Males Ages 18-81	Females Ages 16-52	Males Ages 18-62	Females Ages 18-37	Males Ages 22-57
Acne: indurata	6	4	2	1	..	..
rosacea	7	3	1	1	..	..
vulgaris	5	4	5	2	..	..
Angioneurotic edema: urticaria	3	..	2	1	1	..
Atopic dermatitis	12	5	10	3	..	..
Chronic infectious eczema- toid dermatitis	10	5	11	2	1	..
Contact dermatitis	5	4	5	1	..	1
Dermatitis medicamentosa	2	..	1	..	..	..
Hyperhidrosis	1	1	1	1	..	..
Intertrigo	2	..	3	..	..	..
Lichen planus	3	..	2	..	..	..
Lichen sclerosus et atrophicus	1	..	1	1	..	..
Lupus erythematosus: subacute disseminated	1	..	1	..	..	..
Neurodermatitis	4	1	3	..	..	..
Seborrheic dermatitis	7	3	4	1	1	1
Stasis dermatitis	5	1	3	..	2	..
Totals	74	31	55	14	5	2

Grand Total...............181

The longest interval of treatment was six months: the shortest, 21 days: the average, three months.

For both groups of patients, after four consecutive weeks of therapy, urinalyses and hemograms were obtained for 23 patients. Monthly urinalyses and hemograms were obtained for 27 patients, who received the drug for six months. All chemistries, obtained after the institution of therapy, were compared with those obtained before the start of therapy, and all remained unchanged. There were no instances of hematopoietic, renal or hepatic dysfunction.

None of our patients in either series complained of unpleasant subjective symptoms from Quiactin. A number of patients resumed driving their cars while under therapy. (It was our suggestion that they refrain from doing so, until they found out what effects the new medication would have.) We heard no complaints of drowsiness, sleepiness, or inability to concentrate. Objective symptoms, such as excoriations, pruritus, erythema and extension of lesions showed improvement, which we attributed to the tranquilizing and calming effects of oxanamide. We realize, of course, that no tranquilizing agent affects, specifically, any dermatological problem.

In patients, who had been under therapy with other tranquilizing agents, such as phenothiazines; rauwolfia, fractions and alkaloids; substituted propanediols, and the like, we observed gradual disappearance of all of the unpleasant subjective symptoms of previously-used medications: for example, "tired all of the time," "logginess," "grogginess," "hangover," "don't want to move, just want to sit," nasal congestion, bad dreams and nightmares. The disappearance of these side effects of previous therapy, in some cases, took as long as two to four weeks. (It will be recalled that Rein and Goodman observed that reserpine-effects in their series, extended beyond the period of placebo therapy.[192])

We observed no evidence of addiction and no withdrawal symptoms, when oxanamide therapy was discontinued.

Twenty patients were arbitrarily selected from each group, and without notification (or knowledge) of change in medication, were maintained for a period of three weeks on placebo tablets. During that interval, from 18 patients, we received complaints that "the medicine isn't working so well," and in 16 patients, we observed evidence of increased excoriations and general exacerbation of dermatoses.

We observed that it was seldom necessary to use a daily dosage of oxanamide of more than 1,200 mg. Most of our patients were relaxed and calm, after taking 800 mg. daily. We intend to continue our study, to determine whether or not maintenance can be satisfactory with a single tablet daily, once favorable response has been achieved on higher dosages.

In our experience to date, oxanamide appears to be the only tranquilizing agent which can be administered in high dosages (400 mg. tablets, three or four times daily) during a prolonged interval (as long as six months) without producing any toxic reactions or side effects, such as photosensitivity, dermatitis, allergic phenomena, liver damage, depression and suicidal tendencies, extrapyramidal dysfunction, convulsions or seizures.

From our experience, we conclude at this writing, that oxanamide is the medication of choice for the tranquilization of dermatological patients.

To complete our report, we quote the following statements made by Coats and Gray:[54]

"None of our patients reported disagreeable side effects during the 30-day investigation of Quiactin. There were no instances of excessive drowsiness, stimulation, gastrointestinal disturbance, or withdrawal symptoms following doses of 1.6 Gm. daily. The laboratory tests conducted on each of the patients remained unchanged during and following the test period as compared with the results of the tests before treatment. No hemato-, nephro-, or hepato-toxicity attributable to Quiactin was demonstrated. We were unable to detect any cumulative effects of the drug on the basis of these observations and of our subjective psychiatric evaluations."

Recapitulation and Conclusions

RECAPITULATION AND CONCLUSIONS

According to some reports[267] (and there are many)—three out of every ten prescriptions written in these United States provide for release, to patients, of psychotherapeutic agents for tranquilization: more than one billion meprobamate tablets alone, were ordered by physicians for 160 million Americans in little more than a year: more than ten million persons have been treated with chlorpromazine:[224] hundreds of millions of dollars have been spent: mental hospitals have become more quiet and less congested. Then I ask (as others have asked): what about the anxiety level of our patients? Presumably it has ebbed, but I ask again: has it?

Even though tranquilizing drugs seem to be of no general harm, nonetheless, it has been said that[264] "they constitute a definite threat to the health and even the life of many patients." Individuals who, seemingly, should be "tranquilized," instead, develop the most unusual untoward reactions. Anxious people become depressed enough to commit suicide; calm, easy-going people become hypomanic, or manic; and many other unpleasant and unfavorable responses require intensive treatment and prolonged hospitalization. Skin changes; blood dyscrasias; allergic phenomena; toxic reactions; toxic liver changes; gastrointestinal upheavals; convulsive disorders; complications of pregnancy, such as abortion; problems of addiction and habituation—these are but some of the results of therapy with psychotherapeutic agents for tranquilization.

It is generally agreed that a mild form of anxiety is beneficial to man. It alerts him, and prepares him against external dangers: it enables him to make adjustments, with himself, his fellows, his environment, with little awareness of somatic participation. What happens when we prescribe drugs to take away that anxiety? We destroy, or at least we temporarily check that "divine unrest" which is maximal in man. There is danger that our possession of psychotherapeutic agents, which can bring tranquility, will only drug man into hopeless inertia.

I end this monograph with a repetition of some of the statements with which I began it. It is my belief that tranquilizing agents offer no substitute for accurate diagnosis or adequate medical supervision: they are adjuncts likely to displace, but never to replace some other forms of therapy. Physicians, who prescribe these drugs indiscriminately, are at fault, rather than the drugs themselves.

BIBLIOGRAPHY

1. Achor, R. W. P.; Hanson, N. O., and Gifford, R. W., Jr.: Hypertension treated with Rauwolfia serpentina (whole root) and with reserpine. *J.A.M.A., 159*:841 (Oct. 29) 1955.
2. Idem.: Hypertension treated with Rauwolfia canescens. A comparison with Rauwolfia serpentina. *New England J. Med., 255*:646 (Oct. 4) 1956.
3. Alexander, L.: Chemotherapy of depression. Use of meprobamate combined with benactyzine (2-diethylaminoethyl benzilate) hydrochloride. *J.A.M.A., 166*:1019 (Mar. 1) 1958.
4. Allen, A. G., and Black, A. V.: Near-fatal case of intoxication with meprobamate treated with electrostimulation and levarterenol. *Ohio State M. J., 52*:1303 (Dec.) 1956.
5. Allergic reaction to meprobamate. (Queries & Minor Notes). *J.A.M.A., 163*:795 (Mar. 2) 1957.
6. Altschule, M. D.: Use of chlorpromazine and reserpine in mental disorders. *New England J. Med., 254*:515 (Mar. 15) 1956.
7. Archer, R. H.: A comparative study of promazine and chlorpromazine for hospital management. *Pennsylvania Med. J., 60*:1343 (Oct.) 1957.
8. Asher, L. M.: Use of chlorpromazine in treatment of certain gastrointestinal disturbances: preliminary report. *J.A.M.A., 160*: 1281 (Apr. 14) 1956.
9. Asung, C. L.; Charcowa, A. I., and Villa, A. P.: Effects of a new tranquilizing drug (Nostyn) on the behavior patterns of children recovered from tuberculous meningitis. *Quart. Rev. Sea View Hosp., 16*:80 (July) 1956.
10. Idem.: A study of the nonhypnotic calmative effect of 2-ethylcrotonylurea (Nostyn) in children with behavior problems. *New York State J. Med., 57*:1911 (June 1) 1957.
11. Atkinson, R. P.: Clinical experiences with promazine (Sparine). *Lahey Clin. Bull., 10*:149 (July-Sept.) 1957.
12. Atkinson, S. C., and Carpenter, C. C.: Seborrheic dermatitis—an evaluation of therapy. *J. M. Soc. New Jersey, 53*:520 (Oct.) 1956.
13. Ayd, F. J., Jr.: The treatment of anxiety, agitation and excitement in the aged. *J. Amer. Geriatrics Soc., 5*:92 (Jan.) 1957.

14. Idem.: Treatment of ambulatory and hospitalized psychiatric patients with Trilafon. *Dis. Nerv. System, 18*:394 (Oct.) 1957.
15. Idem.: A clinical report on benactyzine hydrochloride. *New England J. Med., 257*:669 (Oct. 3) 1957.
16. Azima, H.: The effects of Vesprin in mental syndromes. (A preliminary report). *Monographs on Therapy, 2*:203 (Aug.) 1957.
17. Azima, H., and Durost, H.: Comparison of the effects of promazine and chlorpromazine in mental syndromes. *Canad. M.A.J., 77*:671 (Oct. 1) 1957.
18. Bachman, H., and Freund, J.: Use of phenaglycodol for alleviation of nervous tension in patients with tuberculosis. *Am. Pract. & Digest. Treat., 9*:397 (Mar.) 1958.
19. Baer, R. L., and Witten, V. H.: *The Year Book of Dermatology and Syphilology,* 1957-1958 year book series. Chicago, The Year Book Publishers, Inc., 1958, page 147.
20. Barnett, D. A.: Chlorpromazine as masking agent in intestinal obstruction. *J. Oklahoma M. A., 51*:16 (Jan.) 1958.
21. Barraclough, C. A.: Blockade of the release of pituitary gonadotrophin by reserpine. *Fed. Proc., 14*:9 (Mar.) 1955.
22. Idem.: Induction of pseudopregnancy in the rat by reserpine and chlorpromazine. *Anat. Rec., 127*:262 (Feb.) 1957.
23. Barrett, Capt. O'Neill, Jr.: Convulsive seizures after administration of chlorpromazine. *J.A.M.A., 166*:1986 (Apr. 19) 1958.
24. Barsa, J. A., and Kline, N. S.: Treatment of two hundred disturbed psychotics with reserpine. *J.A.M.A., 158*:110 (May 14) 1955.
25. Idem.: Promazine in chronic schizophrenic patients. *Am. J. Psychiat., 113*:654 (Jan.) 1957.
26. Bartholomew, L. G., and Cain, J. C.: Chlorpromazine hepatitis without clinical jaundice. *Proc. Staff Meet. Mayo Clin., 31*:201 (Apr. 4) 1956.
27. Idem.: Abnormal pain following use of chlorpromazine. *J.A.M.A., 163*:733 (Mar. 2) 1957.
28. Bauer, H. G.; Seegers, W.; Krawzoff, M., and McGavack, T. H.: A clinical evaluation of ectylurea (Nostyn). *New York State J. Med., 58*:520 (Feb. 15) 1958.
29. Becker, F. T.; Fredericks, M. G.; Schmid, J. F., and Tuura, J. L.: An evaluation of meprobamate in the management of selected dermatoses. *A.M.A. Arch. Dermat., 77*:406 (Apr.) 1958.
30. Bello, C. T., and Turner, L. W.: Reserpine as an antihypertensive in the outpatient clinic: a double-blind clinical study. *Am. J.*

Med. Sci., 232:194 (Aug.) 1956.

31. Berger, F. M.: The pharmacological properties of 2-methyl-2-n-propyl-1, 3-propanediol dicarbamate (Miltown), a new inter-neuronal blocking agent. *J. Pharmacol. & Exper. Therap., 112*: 413 (Dec.) 1954.

32. Idem.: Miltown, a long-acting mephenesin-like drug. *Fed. Proc., 14*:318 (Mar.) 1955.

33. Berger, F. M.; Hendley, C. D.; Ludwig, B. J., and Lynes, T. E.: Central depressant and anticonvulsant activity of compounds isomeric with 2-methyl-2-n-propyl-1, 3-propanediol dicarbamate (Miltown). *J. Pharmacol. & Exper. Therap., 116*:337 (Mar.) 1956.

34. Bernthsen, A.: Zur Kenntniss des Methylenbleu und Verwendter Farbstosse. *Ber., 16*:2896, 1883.

35. Blood dyscrasias associated with promazine hydrochloride therapy. Report of the Council on Pharmacy and Chemistry. *J.A.M.A., 165*:685 (Oct. 12) 1957.

36. Blood dyscrasias associated with chlorpromazine therapy. Report of the Council on Pharmacy and Chemistry. *J.A.M.A., 160*:287 (Jan. 28) 1956.

37. Bonello, F. J.: Chlorpromazine in general practice. *Internat. Rec. Med. & Gen. Prac. Clin., 169*:197 (Apr.) 1956.

38. Borrus, J. C.: Study of effect of Miltown (2-methyl-2-n-propyl-1, 3-propanediol dicarbamate) on psychiatric states. *J.A.M.A., 157*:1596 (Apr. 30) 1955.

39. Brill, A.: Laryngeal edema and drugs. (Correspondence). *J.A.M.A., 160*:1355 (Apr. 14) 1956.

40. Brooks, G. W.: Experience with the use of chlorpromazine and reserpine in psychiatry: with especial reference to the signifi-cance and management of extrapyramidal dysfunction. *New England J. Med., 254*:1119 (June 14) 1956.

41. Budnick, I. S.; Leiken, S., and Hoeck, L. E.: Effects in the new-born infant of reserpine administered ante partum. *A.M.A. Am. J. Dis. Child., 90*:286 (Sept.) 1955.

42. Cahn, M. M., and Levy, E. J.: Ultraviolet light factor in chlorpro-mazine dermatitis. *A.M.A. Arch. Dermat., 75*:38 (Jan.) 1957.

43. Cahn, M., Levy, E. J., and Hamilton, W. L.: Photosensitivity studies with Vesprin (MC4703). *Monographs on Therapy, 2*:208 (Aug.) 1957.

44. Callahan, D., and Burrell, Z. L., Jr.: Agranulocytosis-iatrogenic

disease. *Am. Pract. & Digest Treat., 8*:1766 (Nov.) 1957.

45. Callaway, J. L., and Olansky, S.: Trimeprazine: an adjuvant in the management of itching dermatoses. *North Carolina Med. J., 18*:320 (Aug.) 1957.

46. Campbell, M. M.: Chlorpromazine dermatitis. (Correspondence). *J.A.M.A., 159*:398 (Sept. 24) 1955.

47. Canary, J. J.; Schaaf, M.; Duffy, B. J., Jr.; and Kyle, L. H.: Effects of oral and intramuscular administration of reserpine in thyrotoxicosis. *New England J. Med., 257*:435 (Sept. 5) 1957.

48. Carmel, W. J., Jr., and Dannenberg, T.: Nonthrombocytopenic purpura due to Miltown (2-methyl-2-n-propyl-1, 3-propanediol dicarbamate). *New England J. Med., 255*:770 (Oct. 18) 1956.

49. Carmichael, L. P.: Serum sickness type of reaction to meprobamate. *J. Florida Med. Assn., 43*:779 (Feb.) 1957.

50. Charet, R.; Brill, B., and Elloso, C.: Coma after Miltown overdosage. *Ann. Int. Med., 45*:1211 (Dec.) 1956.

51. Charpentier, P.; Gailliot, P.; Jacob, R.; Gaudechon, J.; and Buisson, P.: Récherchés sur les dimethylaminopropyl-n phénothiazines substituées. *Compt. rend., 235*:59 (July 7) 1952.

52. Coady, A., and Jewesbury, E. C. O.: A clinical trial of benactyzine hydrochloride ("Suavitil") as a physical relaxant. *Brit. M. J., 1*:485 (Mar. 3) 1956.

53. Coakley, C. S.; Alpert, S., and Boling, J. S.: Circulatory responses during anesthesia of patients on rauwolfia therapy. *J.A.M.A., 161*:1143 (July 21) 1956.

54. Coats, E. W., and Gray, R. W.: Quiactin in treatment of emotional and mental disorders. *Dis. Nerv. System, 18*:191 (May) 1957.

55. Cohen, I. M., and Archer, J. D.: Liver function and hepatic complications in patients receiving chlorpromazine. *J.A.M.A., 159*: 99 (Sept. 10) 1955.

56. Coirault, R.; Schuller, E., and Perier, M.: Un sedatif pour la pratique quotidienne; l'hydroxyzine. *Presse méd., 64*:2239 (Dec. 26) 1956.

57. Collins-Dineen, M.: Meprobamate toxicity—report of a case. *Ohio State M. J., 52*:1304 (Dec.) 1956.

58. Combes, F. C., and Reisch, M.: Contact dermatitis due to chlorpromazine in a dentist. (Correspondence). *J.A.M.A., 159*:807 (Oct. 22) 1955.

59. Corley, B. L., and Brundage, F.: Reaction following ingestion of 400 mg. meprobamate. *California Med., 86*:183 (Mar.) 1957.

60. Cornbleet, T., and Barsky, S.: The role of the tranquilizing drugs (chlorpromazine and rauwolfia derivatives) in dermatology, presented at the 115th Annual Meeting of the Illinois State Medical Society, Chicago, May 19, 1955.

61. Craft, M.: Tranquilizers in mental deficiency: hydroxyzine. *J. Mental Sci., 103*:855 (Oct.) 1957.

62. Crimson, L.: Toxic reaction to Miltown (Equanil). *Gastroenterology, 26*:619 (Nov.) 1956.

63. Davies, E. B.: A new drug to relieve anxiety. *Brit. M. J., 1*:480 (Mar. 3) 1956.

64. Davies, J. I.; Huggins, D. H. M., and Wolkenstein, C. F.: Pacatal in anesthesia; a preliminary report. *Canad. Anaes. Soc. J., 3*:224 (Feb.) 1956.

65. Davis, M. J.: Comment on Stroud, G.: Drug eruptions from Miltown. *Bull. Assn. Military Dermatologists, 6*:19 (Mar.) 1957.

66. DeFeo, V. J., and Reynolds, S. R. M.: Modification of the menstrual cycle in rheusus monkeys by reserpine. *Science, 124*:726 (Oct. 19) 1956.

67. DeFeo, V. J.: Effect of large doses of reserpine on the deciduoma response. *Anat. Rec., 127*:409 (Feb.) 1957.

68. Delay, J.; Deniker, P.; Green, A., and Mordret, M.: Le syndrome excito-moteur provoqué par les médicaments neuroleptiques. *Presse méd., 65*:1771 (Nov. 2) 1957.

69. Dixon, N. M.: Meprobamate, a clinical evaluation. *Ann. N. Y. Acad. Sci., 67*:772 (May 9) 1957.

70. Douglas, A. D. M., and Bates, T. J. N.: Chlorpromazine as a suicidal agent. (Medical Memorandum). *Brit. M. J., 1*:1514 (June 29) 1957.

71. Doyle, A. E.; McQueen, E. G., and Smirk, F. H.: Treatment of hypertension with reserpine, with reserpine in combination with pentapyrrolidinium and with reserpine in combination with veratrum alkaloids. *Circulation, 11*:170 (Feb.) 1955.

72. Dunsmore, R. A.; Dunsmore, L. D.; Bickford, A. F., and Goldman, A.: Meprobamate as adjuvant therapy in hypertension. A preliminary report. *Am. J. M. Sci., 233*:280 (Mar.) 1957.

73. Ectylurea. Report of the Council on Drugs. *J.A.M.A., 164*:1093 (July 6) 1957.

74. Epstein, John H.; Brunsting, L. A.; Petersen, M. C., and Schwartz, B. E.: A study of photosensitivity occurring with chlorpromazine therapy. *J. Invest. Dermat., 28*:329 (May) 1957.

75. Epstein, Stephan, and Rowe, R. J.: Photoallergy and photocross-sensitivity to Phenergan. *J. Invest. Dermat., 29*:319 (Nov.) 1957.

76. Essig, C. F., and Ainslie, J. D.: Addiction to meprobamate. (Correspondence). *J.A.M.A., 164*:1382 (July 20) 1957.

77. Falk, M. S.: Allergic reaction to meprobamate. *A.M.A. Arch. Dermat., 75*:437 (Mar.) 1957.

78. Favre, J. D.: The successful use of 'Equanil' as a basic adjuvant treatment in asthma exhibiting strong emotional factors. Paper read at the Congress of the International Association of Allergists, Florence, Italy, September, 1956.

79. Fazekas, J. F.; Schultz, J. D.; Sullivan, P. D., and Shea, J. G.: Management of acutely disturbed patients with promazine. *J.A.M.A., 161*:46 (May 5) 1956.

80. Feinblatt, T. M.; Feinblatt, H. M., and Ferguson, E. A., Jr.: Rauwolfia-ephedrine as a hypotensive-tranquilizer. *J.A.M.A., 161*: 424 (June 2) 1956.

81. Feldman, P. E.; Bertone, J., and Panthel, H.: Fatal agranulocytosis during treatment with Pacatal. *Am. J. Psychiat., 113*:842 (Mar.) 1957.

82. Feldman, P. E.: Clinical evaluation of Pacatal. *Am. J. Psychiat., 114*:143 (Aug.) 1957.

83. Ferguson, J. T.: Comparison of reserpine and Harmonyl in psychiatric patients. A preliminary report. *Journal-Lancet, 76*:389 (Dec.) 1956.

84. Idem.: Successful therapeutic regimen for the management of behavior problems in the elderly. *J. Am. Geriatrics Soc., 4*:1080 (Nov.) 1956.

85. Idem.: Neuropharmacological agents in rehabilitation of patients with chronic mental illness. A three-year clinical evaluation. *J.A.M.A., 165*:1677 (Nov. 30) 1957.

86. Ferguson, J. T., and Linn, F. V. Z.: A new compound for the symptomatic treatment of tension and anxiety: 2-ethyl-crotonyl-urea (Nostyn). *Antibiotic Med. & Clin. Ther., 3*:329 (Oct.) 1956.

87. Ferrara, R. J., and Pinkus, H.: Alseroxylon in the treatment of pruritic and psychogenic dermatoses. *A.M.A. Arch. Dermat., 72*:23 (July) 1955.

88. Feuss, C. D., and Gragg, L., Jr.: Quiactin: an adjunct in the treatment of chronic psychoses. *Dis. Nerv. System, 18*:29 (Jan.) 1957.

89. Feuss, C. D., Jr., and Ivanov, C. J.: Quiactin as an outpatient drug. *Marquette Med. Rev., 23*:78 (Jan.) 1958.

90. Figurelli, F. A.: Delirium tremens. Reduction of mortality and morbidity with promazine. *J.A.M.A., 166*:747 (Feb. 15) 1958.
91. Finnerty, F. A., and Buchholz, J. H.: The cardiovascular dynamics of Vesprin. *Monographs on Therapy, 2*:210 (Aug.) 1957.
92. Fisher, R. A., and D'Silva, J. L.: Chlorpromazine in the management of psoriasis. *Illinois M. J., 110*:135 (Sept.) 1956.
93. Flipse, M. J.: Pacatal in office practice. *Clin. Med. 4*: No. 10 (Oct.) 1957.
94. Ford, R. V., and Moyer, J. H.: Rauwolfia toxicity in the treatment of hypertension: comparative toxicity of reserpine and alseroxylon. *Postgrad. Med., 23*:41 (Jan.) 1958.
95. Freed, H.: Some preliminary observations on the use of Vesprin in children and adults. *Monographs on Therapy, 2*:197 (Aug.) 1957.
96. Freis, E. D.: Mental depression in hypertensive patients treated for long periods with large doses of reserpine. *New England J. Med., 251*:1006 (Dec. 16) 1954.
97. Friedman, H. T., and Marmelzat, W. L.: Adverse reactions to meprobamate. *J.A.M.A., 162*:628 (Oct. 13) 1956.
98. Gallagher, W. J., and Pfeiffer, C. C.: One year of Vesprin therapy in chronic schizophrenia. *Monographs on Therapy, 2*:188 (Aug.) 1957.
99. Gambescia, J.; Imbriglia, J.; Galamaga, P., and Winkelman, W.: Jaundice associated with the administration of chlorpromazine. *Gastroenterology, 30*:735 (May) 1956.
100. Gaunt, R. A.; Renzi, A.; Antonchak, N.; Miller, G. J., and Gilman, M.: Endocrine aspects of the pharmacology of reserpine. *Ann. N. Y. Acad. Sci., 59*:22 (Apr. 30) 1954.
101. Gillie, A. K.: The use of Pacatal in low-grade mental defectives. *J. Mental Sci., 103*:402 (Apr.) 1957.
102. Goldman, D.: Observations on the clinical use of Vesprin. *Monographs on Therapy, 2*:177 (Aug.) 1957.
103. Gore, C. P., and Walton, D.: Benactyzine in the treatment of anxiety and tension. (Letters to the Editor). *Lancet, 2*:294 (Aug. 10) 1957.
104. Gottlieb, F. I.: Tranquilizers and purpura hemorrhagica. (Correspondence). *J.A.M.A., 161*:96 (May 5) 1956.
105. Grandon, R. C.; Heffley, W.; Hensel, T., and Bashore, S.: A new medical adjunct to the treatment of alcoholism: the use of reserpine (Serpasil). *Am. Pract. & Digest Treat., 7*:231 (Feb.) 1956.

106. Gray, W. D.: An appraisal of a new antiemetic drug: prochlorperazine. *Internat. Rec. Med. & Gen. Pract. Clin., 170*:469 (Aug.) 1957.

107. Grenell, R. G.; Mendelson, J., and McElroy, W. D.: Effects of chlorpromazine on metabolism in the central nervous system. *Arch. Neurol. & Psychiat., 73*:347 (Mar.) 1955.

108. Gruber, C. H., Jr., and Mosier, J. M.: Phenaglycodol: a new antiepileptic agent. *Proc. Soc. Exper. Biol. & Med., 94*:384 (Feb.) 1957.

109. Gunter, M. J.: Convulsive seizures following administration of chlorpromazine (Thorazine). *Ohio State M. J., 54*:51 (Jan.) 1958.

110. Hargreaves, G. R.; Hamilton, M., and Roberts, J. M.: Benactyzine as an aid in treatment of anxiety states. Preliminary report. *Brit. M. J., 1*:306 (Feb. 9) 1957.

111. Harris, R. D., and Rowley, E. H.: Reserpine in cerebral palsy. *J. Pediat., 49*:398 (Oct.) 1956.

112. Heberden, P., and Cooper, W.: Attempted suicide with meprobamate treated with Leptazol. *Brit. M. J., 1*:1513 (June 29) 1957.

113. Herschberger, R. L.; Dennis, E. W., and Moyer, J. H.: The response to rescinnamine administered parenterally and orally for the treatment of hypertension. *Am. J. Med. Sci., 231*:542 (May) 1956.

114. Hiles, B. W.: Hyperglycemia, and glycosuria following chlorpromazine therapy. (Correspondence). *J.A.M.A., 162*:1651 (Dec. 29) 1956.

115. Hodges, H. H., and LaZerte, G. D.: Jaundice and agranulocytosis with fatality following chlorpromazine therapy. (Clinical Notes). *J.A.M.A., 158*:114 (May 14) 1955.

116. Hollister, L. E.; Stannard, A. N., and Drake, C. F.: Treatment of anxious patients with drugs. *Dis. Nerv. System, 17*:289 (Sept.) 1956.

117. Hollister, L. E.: Allergy to chlorpromazine manifested by jaundice. *Am. J. Med., 23*:870 (Dec.) 1957.

118. Holmes, C. R., and Stone, H. M.: Agranulocytosis due to chlorpromazine: report of a case with recovery. *J. South Carolina M. A., 52*:42 (Feb.) 1956.

119. Hubbard, B. A., Jr.: Reserpine. (Correspondence). *J.A.M.A., 157*:468 (Jan. 29) 1955.

120. Hughes, W. M.; Moyer, J. H., and Daeschner, W. C., Jr.: Paren-

teral reserpine in treatment of hypertensive emergencies. *A.M.A. Arch. Int. Med., 95*:563 (Apr.) 1955.

121. Hutcheon, D. E.; Scriabine, A., and Morris, D. L.: Cardiovascular action of hydroxyzine (Atarax). *J. Pharmacol. & Exper. Therap., 118*:451 (Dec.) 1956.

122. Hydroxyzine hydrochloride. Report of the Council on Pharmacy and Chemistry. *J.A.M.A., 162*:205 (Sept. 15) 1956.

123. Impotence and reserpine therapy. (Queries & Minor Notes). *J.A.M.A., 163*:909 (Mar. 9) 1957.

124. Irwin, S., and Govier, W. M.: Perphenazine (Trilafon), a new potent tranquilizer and antiemetic. (In press).

125. Isaacs, B., and Macarthur, J. G.: Influence of chlorpromazine and promethazine on vomiting induced with apomorphine in man. *Lancet, 2*:570 (Sept. 18) 1954.

126. Isaacs, B.; Macarthur, J. G., and Taylor, R. M.: Jaundice in relation to chlorpromazine therapy. *Brit. M. J., 2*:1122 (Nov. 5) 1955.

127. Karlinsky, W.: Allergic purpura due to meprobamate. (Letter.) *Canadian M. A. J., 74*:1012 (June 15) 1956.

128. Kass, I., and Brown, E. C.: Treatment of hypertensive patients with rauwolfia compounds and reserpine. Depressive and psychotic changes. *J.A.M.A., 159*:1513 (Dec. 17) 1955.

129. Kelsey, J. R., Jr.: Moyer, J. H.; Brown, W. G., and Bennett, H. D.: Chlorpromazine jaundice. *Gastroenterology, 29*:865 (Nov.) 1955.

130. Kinross-Wright, V.: Intensive chlorpromazine treatment of schizophrenia. *Psychiat. Research Rep., 1*:53 (Jan.) 1955.

131. Kinross-Wright, V., and Moyer, J. H.: Observations upon the therapeutic use of benactyzine (Suavitil). (Clinical Notes). *Am. J. Psychiat., 114*:73 (July) 1957.

132. Klotz, S. D., and Bernstein, C.: Allergy to meprobamate with some observations regarding tranquilizing drugs. *Southern M. J., 50*:1478 (Dec.) 1957.

133. Knapp, M. R., and Beecher, H. K.: Postanesthetic nausea, vomiting, and retching. *J.A.M.A., 160*:376 (Feb. 4) 1956.

134. Koetschet, P.: Can it be said that chlorpromazine has specific properties? *Internat. Rec. Med. & Gen. Pract. Clin., 168*:295 (May) 1955.

135. Kohl, G. C.; Maddison, F. R., and Davis, R. E.: Jaundice after discontinuance of chlorpromazine. *Northwest. Med., 54*:716 (July) 1955.

136. Kositchek, R. J.: Reactions to meprobamate. (Correspondence.) *J.A.M.A., 161*:644 (June 16) 1956.

137. Kurtzke, J. F.: Seizures with promazine. Preliminary report. *J. Nerv. & Mental Dis., 125*:119 (Jan.-Mar.) 1957.

138. Lemere, F.: Drug habituation. (Correspondence). *J.A.M.A., 160*:1431 (Apr. 21) 1956.

139. Idem.: Habit-forming properties of meprobamate (Miltown or Equanil). *A.M.A. Arch. Neurol. & Psychiat., 76*:205 (Aug.) 1956.

140. Lemire, R. E., and Mitchell, R. A.: Regurgitation type of jaundice during prolonged therapy with chlorpromazine. *A.M.A. Arch. Int. Med., 95*:840 (June) 1955.

141. Leslie, G.: Rauwolfia serpentina in the treatment of psoriasis. *Monographs on Therapy, 1*:29 (Jan.) 1956.

142. Lesse, S.: An evaluation of prochlorperazine in the ambulatory treatment of psychiatric patients. *Internat. Rec. Med. & Gen. Pract. Clin., 170*:599 (Oct.) 1957.

143. Levan, N. E.: Meprobamate reaction. *A.M.A. Arch. Dermat., 75*:437 (Mar.) 1957.

144. Levan, P., and Wright, E. T.: Use of tranquilizers in diseases of the skin: a preliminary report. *California Med., 85*:87 (Aug.) 1956.

145. Lewis, G. M., and Sawicky, H. H.: Contact dermatitis from chlorpromazine. Report of two cases. *J.A.M.A., 157*:909 (Mar. 12) 1955.

146. Locket, S.: Oral preparations of Rauwolfia serpentina in treatment of essential hypertension. *Brit. M. J., 1*:809 (Apr. 2) 1955.

147. Lockhart, W. E.: Suicidal Miltown, hazard of overhydration in treatment. *Southwestern Med., 37*:428 (July) 1956.

148. Lomas, J.: Chlorpromazine and agranulocytosis. (Correspondence). *Brit. M. J., 2*:358 (Aug. 7) 1954.

149. Lomas, J.; Boardman, R. H., and Markowe, M.: Complications of chlorpromazine therapy in 800 mental-hospital patients. *Lancet, 1*:1144 (June 4) 1955.

150. McAfoos, L. G., Jr.: Prochlorperazine (Compazine) in emotional disturbances. *Dis. Nerv. System, 18*:430 (Nov.) 1957.

151. McGee, R. R.: Drug reaction. (Correspondence.) *J.A.M.A., 161*:1094 (July 14) 1956.

152. McHardy, G.; McHardy, R., and Canale, S.: Chlorpromazine (Thorazine) hepatitis. *Gastroenterology, 29*:184 (Aug.) 1955.

153. McNeill, J. F.; Johnston, W. C., and Pietuchow, W.: Serpasil in a

hospital for the mentally ill with criminal tendencies. *New York J. Med.,* 56:1911 (June 15) 1956.

154. McQueen, E. G.; Doyle, A. E., and Smirk, F. H.: The circulatory effects of reserpine. *Circulation,* 11:161 (Feb.) 1955.

155. Marangoni, B. A.: Use of a new tranquilizer, perphenazine, in 60 patients with anxiety and tension. *Am. Pract. & Digest Treat.,* 8:1959 (Dec.) 1957.

156. Margolis, L. H.; Butler, R. N., and Fischer, A.: Nonrecurring chlorpromazine dermatitis. *A.M.A. Arch. Dermat.,* 72:72 (July) 1955.

157. Mauceri, J., and Strauss, H.: Effects of chlorpromazine on electroencephalogram, with report of a case of chlorpromazine intoxication. *Electroencephalog. & Clin. Neurophysiol.,* 8:671 (Nov.) 1956.

158. May, R. H., and Voegele, G. E.: Parkinsonian reactions following chlorpromazine and reserpine: similar reactions in the same patients. *A.M.A. Arch. Neurol. & Psychiat.,* 75:522 (May) 1956.

159. Melby, J. C.; Street, J. P., and Watson, C. J.: Chlorpromazine in the treatment of porphyria. *J.A.M.A.,* 162:174 (Sept. 15) 1956.

160. Mitchell, E. H.: Treatment of acute alcoholism with promazine (Sparine). *J.A.M.A.,* 161:44 (May 5) 1956.

161. Monaco, R. N.; Leeper, R. D.; Robbins, J. J., and Calvy, G. L.: Intermittent acute porphyria treated with chlorpromazine. *New England J. Med.,* 256:309 (Feb. 14) 1957.

162. Movitt, E. R.; Meyer, M. A.; Snell, A. M.; Goldman, M. J.; Gibson, Maj. J. R.; Sullivan, Col. B. H., Jr.; Webster, J. G., and Stone, R. B.: Jaundice associated with administration of chlorpromazine. S. K. F. 2601A (Thorazine). Report of three cases, with biopsies of the liver. *Gastroenterology,* 28:901 (June) 1955.

163. Moyer, J. H.; Kinard, S. A.; Herschberger, R., and Dennis, E. W.: Desperidine (canescine) for the treatment of hypertension. *Southern M. J.,* 50:499 (Apr.) 1957.

164. Muller, J. C.; Pryor, W. W.; Gibbons, J. E., and Orgain, E. S.: Depression and anxiety occurring during rauwolfia therapy. *J.A.M.A.,* 159:836 (Oct. 29) 1955.

165. Mullins, J. F.; Cohen, I. M., and Farrington, E. S.: Cutaneous sensitivity reactions to chlorpromazine. *J.A.M.A.,* 162:946 (Nov. 3) 1956.

166. *New and Nonofficial Drugs,* containing descriptions of therapeutic, prophylactic and diagnostic agents evaluated by the Council

on Drugs (formerly Council on Pharmacy and Chemistry) of the American Medical Association. Philadelphia, J. B. Lippincott Co., 1958.

167. Newman, B. A.: The changing pattern of drug eruptions. Presidential address, Pacific Dermatological Association Meeting, Phoenix, Arizona, November, 1957.

168. Nielsen, R. H.: The use of perphenazine in ocular surgery. A preliminary report. *Am. J. Ophth.* (In press).

169. Nieschulz, O.; Popendiker, K., and Sack, K.: Pharmakologische Untersuchungen über N-Alkly-piperidyl-phenothiazinderivate. *Arzneimitt.-Forsch., 4:*232 (April) 1954.

170. Nieschulz, O.; Popendiker, K., and Hoffman, I.: Weitere Pharmakologische Untersuchungen über N-methyl-piperidyl-(3)-methyl phenothiazin. *Arzneimitt.-Forsch., 5:*680 (Dec.) 1955.

171. Niswander, G. D.; Lind, S., and Schlesinger, J.: Vesprin in the treatment of mental illness. *Monographs on Therapy, 2:*184 (Aug.) 1957.

172. Ostergaard, J. O.: Benactyzinterapi ved Psychoneuroser. *Nord. Med., 57:*428 (Mar. 21) 1957.

173. Panaccio, V.: L'action de la resérpine dans certaines affections dermatologiques. *Union Méd. Canada, 84:*672 (June) 1955.

174. Pelner, L.: Meprobamate. (Correspondence.) *J.A.M.A., 162:*137 (Sept. 8) 1956.

175. Pelner, L., and Waldman, S.: Chlorpromazine-induced jaundice. *Postgrad. Med., 18:*349 (Oct.) 1955.

176. Pepin, J. M.; Therien, B.; Vitye, B.; Lemieux, G., and Genest, J.: Treatment of arterial hypertension with recanescine. *Canad. M. A. J., 76:*486 (Mar. 15) 1957.

177. Perera, G. A.: Edema and congestive failure related to administration of Rauwolfia serpentine. *J.A.M.A., 159:*439 (Oct. 1) 1955.

178. Perrot, R. M.; Moreau-Gaudry, G., and LeBorgne, Y.: Manifestations cardiques d'hypokalièmie dans la cure a la chlorpromazine. *Presse méd., 64:*2076 (Dec. 12) 1956.

179. Piala, J. J.; Hassert, G. L., Jr.; High, J. P., and Burke, J. C.: Pharmacology of Vesprin. *Monographs on Therapy, 2:*214 (Aug.) 1957.

180. Pillsbury, D. M.; Shelley, W. B.; Hambrick, G. W.; Hamilton, W. L., and Messenger, A. L.: Experience of the University of Pennsylvania group with trimeprazine (Temaril). *The Schoch*

Letter (November) 1957.

181. Pindell, M. H.; Fancher, O. E., and Lim, R. K. S.: Sedative-hypnotic properties of 2-ethylcrotonylurea. *Fed. Proc., 12*:357 (Mar.) 1953.

182. Pletscher, A.; Shore, P. A., and Brodie, B. B.: Serotonin release as a possible mechanism of reserpine action. *Science, 122*:374 (Aug. 26) 1955.

183. Plummer, A. J.; Earl, A.; Schneider, J. A.; Trapold, J., and Barrett, W.: Pharmacology of rauwolfia alkaloids, including reserpine. *Ann. N. Y. Acad. Sci., 59*:8 (Apr. 30) 1954.

184. Potential hazards of meprobamate. Report of the Council on Pharmacy and Chemistry. *J.A.M.A., 164*:1332 (July 20) 1957.

185. Prescod, H. J., and Townley, M. C.: Management of chronically disturbed patients with sparine. *J. Michigan State Med. Soc., 56*:1273 (Oct.) 1957.

186. Prochlorperazine. Report of the Council on Drugs. *J.A.M.A., 167*:468 (May 24) 1958.

187. Proctor, R. C.: A part-time psychiatric program for a moderate-sized industry. *Dis. Nerv. System, 18*:102 (June) 1957.

188. Purkis, I. E.: Potentiation of obstetric analgesia with **Pacatal.** *Canad. M. A. J., 78*:245 (Feb.) 1958.

189. Rahill, M. A.: Mammary gland changes during chlorpromazine therapy. (Medical Memorandum.) *Brit. M. J., 2*:806 (Oct. 5) 1957.

190. Raymer, W. J.: Discussion on Klotz, S. D., and Bernstein, C.: Allergy to meprobamate with some observations regarding tranquilizing drugs. *Southern M. J., 50*:1478 (Dec.) 1957.

191. Raymond, M. J., and Lucas, C. J.: Benactyzine in psychoneurosis with a note on the E. E. G. changes in normal subjects. *Brit. M. J., 1*:952 (Apr. 28) 1956.

192. Rein, C. R., and Goodman, J. J.: The tranquilizing efficacy of reserpine in dermatological therapy. *Ann. N. Y. Acad. Sci., 61*: 230 (Apr. 15) 1955.

193. Reserpine. Report of the Council on Pharmacy and Chemistry. *J.A.M.A., 159*:1206 (Nov. 19) 1955.

194. Richards, R. W.: Rauwolfia, B. P. C. Renewed interest in an old Indian remedy. *Mfg. Chemist, 25*:253 (June) 1954.

195. Robinson, H. M., Jr.; Robinson, R. C. V., and Strahan, J. F.: Hydroxyzine (Atarax) hydrochloride in dermatological therapy. *J.A.M.A., 161*:604 (June 16) 1956.

196. Idem.: Hydroxyzine hydrochloride (Atarax): a new tranquilizer. *Southern M. J., 50*:1282 (Oct.) 1957.

197. Rogers, S. F.: Reserpine and the newborn infant. (Correspondence.) *J.A.M.A., 160*:1090 (Mar. 24) 1956.

198. Rosenthal, M., and O'Donnell, A. E.: Agranulocytosis due to chlorpromazine. *Ohio State M. J., 53*:1424 (Dec.) 1957.

199. Ross, M. S.: Drug eruption from Rauwolfia serpentina. *A. M. A. Arch. Dermat., 75*:439 (Mar.) 1957.

200. Ross, W. D.: Mistakes in the use of chlorpromazine. *Ohio State M. J., 53*:182 (Feb.) 1957.

201. St. James, A. T., and Ryan, A. J.: Reserpine therapy producing massive gastric and duodenal hemorrhage. *Connecticut M. J., 21*:418 (May) 1957.

202. Sainz, A. A.: The management of side effects of chlorpromazine and reserpine. *Psychiat. Quart., 30*:647 (Oct.) 1956.

203. Samuels, A. S.: Acute chlorpromazine poisoning. *Am. J. Psychiat., 113*:746 (Feb.) 1957.

204. Schick, G., and Virks, J.: Agranulocytosis associated with chlorpromazine therapy. Report of a case and review of the literature. *New England J. Med., 255*:798 (Oct. 25) 1956.

205. Schmidt, K.: Thrombopenia during treatment with reserpine. (Foreign Letters.) *J.A.M.A., 162*:227 (Sept. 15) 1956.

206. Schoch, A. G.: Fixed drug eruptions due to meprobamate. *The Schoch Letter* (January) 1957.

207. Schreader, C. J., and Etzl, M. M.: Premature ventricular contractions due to rauwolfia therapy. (Correspondence.) *J.A.M.A., 162*:1256 (Nov. 24) 1956.

208. Schroeder, H. A., and Perry, H. M., Jr.: Psychosis apparently produced by reserpine. *J.A.M.A., 159*:839 (Oct. 29) 1955.

209. Schultz, K. H.; Wiskemann, A., and Wulf, K.: Klinische und experimentelle Untersuchungen über die Photodynamische Wirksamkeit von Phenothiazin Derivaten, insbesondere von Megaphen. *Arch. f. klin. u. exper. Dermat., 202*:285 (Feb.) 1956.

210. Schwartz, F. R.: Ultran as a dermatological tranquilizer. *Illinois M. J., 112*:273 (Dec.) 1957.

211. Scott, P. A. L.; Grimshaw, L., and Molony, H. M. P.: Hypotensive episodes following treatment with meprobamate. (Correspondence.) *Lancet, 2*:1158 (Dec. 1) 1956.

212. Selling, L. S.: Clinical study of a new tranquilizing drug: use of Miltown (2-methyl-2-n-propyl-1, 3-propanediol dicarbamate).

J.A.M.A., 157:1594 (Apr. 30) 1955.

213. Idem.: A clinical study of Miltown, a new tranquilizing agent. *J. Clin. & Exper. Psychopath. & Quart. Rev. Psychiat. & Neurol., 17*:7 (Jan.-Mar.) 1956.

214. Seneca, H.: Hydroxyzine (Atarax) as a therapeutic agent. *Antibiotic Med. & Clin. Ther., 4*:25 (Jan.) 1957.

215. Settel, E.: Clinical observations on the use of hydroxyzine in anxiety-tension states and senile agitation. *Am. Pract. & Digest Treat., 8*:1584 (Oct.) 1957.

216. Idem.: Phenaglycodol for geriatric agitation. *Geriatrics, 12*:607 (Oct.) 1957.

217. Seville, R. H.: Chlorpromazine dermatitis in nurses. *Brit. J. Dermat., 68*:332 (Oct.) 1956.

218. Shane, A. M., and Hirsch, S.: Three cases of meprobamate poisoning. *Canad. M. A. J., 74*:908 (June 1) 1956.

219. Shannon, J.; David, E., and Haim, O.: Nonrecurring athrombocytopenic purpura after chlorpromazine. *Dermatologica, 114*:101 (Feb.) 1957.

220. Shanon, J.: A dermatologic and psychiatric study of perphenazine (Trilafon) in dermatology. *A. M. A. Arch. Dermat., 77*:119 (Jan.) 1958.

221. Side-effects of reserpine. (Queries & Minor Notes.) *J.A.M.A., 163*:1418 (Apr. 13) 1957.

222. Slater, I. H.; Jones, G. T., and Young, W. K.: Mode of action of phenaglycodol, a new neurosedative agent. *Proc. Soc. Exp. Biol. & Med., 93*:528 (Dec.) 1956.

223. Smirk, F. H., and McQueen, E. G.: Comparison of rescinnamine and reserpine as hypotensive agents. *Proc. Univ. of Otago Med. School, 33*:10 (Apr. 28) 1955.

224. Smith Kline & French Laboratories: *Thorazine Reference Manual.* Philadelphia, 3rd ed. (March) 1958.

225. Smith, R. T.; Hermann, I. F.; Kron, K. M., and Peak, W. P.: Meprobamate (Miltown) in rheumatic diseases. *J.A.M.A., 163*:535 (Feb. 16) 1957.

226. Sokoloff, O. J.: Meprobamate (Miltown) as adjunct in treatment of anogenital pruritus. *A. M. A. Arch. Dermat. & Syph., 74*:393 (Oct.) 1956.

227. Sprogis, G. R.; Lezdins, V.; White, S. D.; Ming, C.; Lanning, M. D.; Miles, E., and Wyckoff, G.: Comparative study on Thorazine and Serpasil in the mental defective. *Am. J. Mental Def.,*

61:737 (Oct.) 1957.

228. Stein, A. A., and Wright, A. W.: Hepatic pathology in jaundice due to chlorpromazine. *J.A.M.A., 161*:508 (June 9) 1956.

229. Stroud, G. M.: Drug eruptions due to meprobamate. *New England J. Med., 256*:354 (Feb. 21) 1957.

230. Idem.: Drug eruptions from Miltown. Bull. Assn. *Military Dermatologists, 6*:19 (Mar.) 1957.

231. Sullivan, C. L.: Prochlorperazine for the treatment of nausea and vomiting of early pregnancy. *New England J. Med., 258*:232 (Jan. 30) 1958.

232. Sussman, R. M., and Sumner, P.: Jaundice following administration of 50 mg. chlorpromazine. *New England J. Med., 253*:499 (Sept. 22) 1955.

233. Sweeney, J. E.: Acute intermittent porphyria. Report of a case treated with chlorpromazine. *J. Kansas M. Soc., 58*:665 (Oct.) 1957.

234. Sympathetic suppressant. *M. D., 2*:62 (May) 1958.

235. Tasker, J. R.: Fatal agranulocytosis during treatment with chlorpromazine. *Brit. M. J., 1*:950 (Apr. 16) 1955.

236. Tilley, R. F., and Barry, H., Jr.: Chlorpromazine treatment for relief of itching in severe and refractory neurodermatitis. *New England J. Med., 252*:229 (Feb. 10) 1955.

237. Trethowan, W. H., and Scott, P. A. L.: Chlorpromazine in obsessive-compulsive and allied disorders. *Lancet, 1*:781 (Apr. 16) 1955.

238. Turrell, R.: Modern treatment of pruritis ani. *Surg. Gynec. & Obst., 104*:233 (Feb.) 1957.

239. Usdin, G. L.: Use of promazine in psychiatric practice; an early study. *J. Louisiana State M. Soc., 108*:251 (July) 1956.

240. Van Gasse, J. J.: Counseling and ataraxia: an effective combination in the management of alcoholics. *Clin. Med., 5*:No. 2 (Feb.) 1958.

241. Van Omnen, R. A., and Brown, C. H.: Obstructive-type jaundice due to chlorpromazine (Thorazine). Report of three cases. *J.A.M.A., 157*:321 (Jan. 22) 1955.

242. Velardo, J. T.: Induction of pseudopregnancy in adult rats with Trilafon, a highly potent tranquilizer of low toxicity. *Fertility & Sterility, 9*:60 (Jan.-Feb.) 1958.

243. Voegele, G. E., and May, R. H.: Epileptiform seizures under promazine therapy: occurrence in two cases without history of former seizures. *Am. J. Psychiat., 113*:655 (Jan.) 1957.

244. Warren, M. R.; Thompson, C. R., and Werner, H. W.: Pharmacological studies on the hypnotic, 2-ethyl-3-propylglycidamide. *J. Pharmacol. & Exper. Therap.*, *96*:209 (June) 1949.

245. Watkins, W. T., Jr.: Discussion on Robinson, R. C. V., and Robinson, H. M., Jr.: Control of emotional tension in dermatoses. *Southern M. J.*, *51*:509 (Apr.) 1958.

246. *Idem.*: Personal communication.

247. Watson, C. J.: Porphyria. *J.A.M.A.*, *164*:1424 (July 20) 1957.

248. Wax, D. S., and DeGraff, A. C.: Clinical study of hypotensive and sedative effects of oral chlorpromazine therapy in cardiovascular disease. *J. Am. Geriatrics Soc.*, *4*:151 (Feb.) 1956.

249. Welsh, A. L.: *The Dermatologist's Handbook.* Springfield, Thomas, 1957, page 191.

250. Welsh, A. L., and Ede, M.: Experience with benactyzine hydrochloride (Suavitil) in dermatologic practice. *A. M. A. Arch. Dermat.*, *76*:466 (Oct.) 1957.

251. Whitelaw, M. J.: Delay in ovulation and menstruation induced by chlorpromazine. *J. Clin. Endocrinol.*, *16*:972 (July) 1956.

252. Williamson, P.: Office treatment of atopic dermatitis. *M. Times*, *84*:1086 (Oct.) 1956.

253. Wilson, B. N., and Wimberley, N. A., Jr.: Production of premature ventricular contractions by rauwolfia. *J.A.M.A.*, *159*:1363 (Dec. 3) 1955.

254. Winton, S. S.: Therapeutic value and limitations of an ataractic drug, (rescinnamine). Internat. *Rec. Med. & Gen. Pract. Clin.*, *170*:665 (Dec.) 1957.

255. Witherspoon, F. G.: Toxic purpura from meprobamate. *Am. Pract. & Digest Treat.*, *8*:270 (Feb.) 1957.

256. Woodward, D. J., and Solomon, J. D.: Fatal agranulocytosis occurring during promazine (Sparine) therapy. *J.A.M.A.*, *162*:1308 (Dec. 1) 1956.

257. Yale, H. L.: The development of a new ataractic agent, Vesprin, 10-(3-dimethylaminopropyl)-2-(trifluoromethyl) phenothiazine hydrochloride, and related compounds. *Monographs on Therapy*, *2*:228 (Aug.) 1957.

258. Zarowitz, H., and Friedman, I. S.: Jaundice following small amounts of chlorpromazine. *New York J. Med.*, *57*:1922 (June 1) 1957.

259. Zeller, W. W.; Graffagnino, P. N.; Cullen, C. F., and Reitman, H. J.: Use of chlorpromazine and reserpine in the treatment of emotional disorders. *J.A.M.A.*, *160*:179 (Jan. 21) 1956.

REVIEWS, EDITORIALS AND COMMENTS

260. Ayd, F. J., Jr.: Tranquilizing drugs in private practice. *New York State J. Med., 57*:1742 (May 15) 1957.
261. Berger, F. M.: The chemistry and mode of action of tranquilizing drugs. *Ann. N. Y. Acad. Sci., 67*:685 (May 9) 1957.
262. Bernstein, C., and Klotz, S. D.: Allergenicity of tranquilizing drugs. *J.A.M.A., 163*:930 (Mar. 16) 1957.
263. Bowes, H. A.: The ataractic drugs: the present position of chlorpromazine, Frenquel, Pacatal and reserpine in the psychiatric hospital. Paper read before the American Psychiatric Association, Chicago, May 4, 1956.
264. Dickel, H. A., and Dixon, H. H.: Inherent dangers in use of tranquilizing drugs in anxiety states. *J.A.M.A., 163*:422 (Feb. 9) 1957.
265. Eisenberg, B. C.: Role of tranquilizing drugs in allergy. *J.A.M.A., 63*:934 (Mar. 16) 1957.
266. Fazekas, J. F.; Shea, J. G.; Ehrmantraut, W. R., and Alman, R. W.: Convulsant action of the phenothiazine derivatives. *J.A.M.A., 165*:1241 (Nov. 9) 1957.
267. Gerard, R. W.: Drugs for the soul: the rise of psychopharmacology. *Science, 125*:201 (Feb. 1) 1957.
268. Goldman, D.: The results of treatment of psychotic states with newer phenothiazine compounds effective in small doses. *Am. J. Med. Sci., 235*:67 (Jan.) 1958.
269. Hollister, L. E.: Medical progress: complications from use of tranquilizing drugs. *New England J. Med., 257*:170 (July 25) 1957.
270. Kinross-Wright, V.: New horizons in the chemotherapy of mental disease. *South African Med. J., 31*:1167 (Nov. 16) 1957.
271. Kurtz, P. L.: The current status of the tranquilizing drugs. *Canad. M. A. J., 78*:209 (Feb. 1) 1958.
272. Lear, E.; Pallin, I. M.; Chiron, A. E.; Rousseau, L., and Aochi, O.: Comparative studies of tranquilizers used in anesthesia. *J.A.M.A., 166*:1438 (Mar. 22) 1958.
273. Moser, Maj. R. H.: Diseases of medical progress. *New England J. Med., 255*:606 (Sept. 27) 1956.
274. Moyer, J. H.; Pevey, K., and Kinross-Wright, V.: Tranquilizing (ataractic) agents: current evaluation of their clinical use in

patients who are not hospitalized. *GP, 15*:97 (June) 1957.

275. Moyer, J. H.; Pevey, K.; Heider, C., and Kinross-Wright, V.: A comparative study of four tranquilizing agents, phenobarbital and inert placebo. *Geriatrics, 13*:153 (Mar.) 1958.

276. Physiologic and pharmacologic basis for the chemotherapy of psychiatric states. (Editorial.) *Am. J. Med., 21*:825 (Dec.) 1956.

277. Psychotherapeutic drugs. Report of the Council on Drugs. *J.A.M.A., 166*:1040 (Mar. 1) 1958.

278. Robinson, R. C. V., and Robinson, H. M., Jr.: Control of emotional tension in dermatoses. *Southern M. J., 51*:509 (Apr.) 1958.

INDEX

Administration, methods of
  (*See* drug, by generic name)
Allergic phenomena
  (*See* drug, by generic name)
Alseroxylon, 58, 62, 70
  (*See* Rauwolfia, reserpine)
Atarax
  (*See* Hydroxyzine hydrochloride)

Benactyzine hydrochloride, 89
  administration, methods of, 90
  clinical uses, general, 91
    dermatological uses, specific, 91
  dosage, 90, 92
  pharmacologic actions, 89
  toxic effects and side reactions:
    allergic phenomena, 92, 94
    cardiovascular complications, 92, 94
    central nervous system effects, 92, 94
    dermal reactions, 93, 94
    endocrine imbalances, 93, 95
    gastrointestinal disturbances, 92, 95

Cardiovascular complications
  (*See* drug, by generic name)
Central nervous system effects
  (*See* drug, by generic name)
Chlorpromazine hydrochloride, 3
  administration, methods of, 5, 7
  clinical uses, general, 5
    dermatological uses, specific, 6
  dosage, 5, 7, 16
  pharmacologic actions, 4
  toxic effects and side reactions:
    allergic phenomena, 13
    cardiovascular complications, 14
    central nervous system effects, 14
    dermal reactions, 8, 16
    endocrine imbalances, 15
    gastrointestinal disturbances, 15
    hematopoietic changes, 15
Clinical uses, general
  (*See* drug, by generic name)

Compazine
  (*See* Prochlorperazine)

Dermal reactions
  (*See* drug, by generic name)
Dermatological uses, specific
  (*See* drug, by generic name)
Dosage
  (*See* drug, by generic name)

Ectylurea, 103
  administration, methods of, 103
  clinical uses, general, 103
    dermatologic uses, specific, 105
  dosage, 103
  pharmacologic actions, 103
  toxic effects and side reactions:
    central nervous system effects,
      104-106
    dermal reactions, 106
    gastrointestinal disturbances, 104, 106
Endocrine imbalances
  (*See* drug, by generic name)
Equanil
  (*See* Meprobamate)

Gastrointestinal disturbances
  (*See* drug, by generic name)

Harmonyl
  (*See* Recanescine)
Hematopoietic changes
  (*See* drug, by generic name)
Hydroxyzine hydrochloride, 95
  administration, methods of, 97
  clinical uses, general, 97
    dermatological uses, specific, 98
  dosage, 97-98, 100
  pharmacologic actions, 96
  toxic effects and side reactions:
    allergic phenomena, 99-100
    central nervous system effects, 98-100
    dermal reactions, 99-100
    gastrointestinal disturbances, 98-100

156